Evangelia,

I h[...]
book as much as I did!
May it inspire you to dance
with all of your body + soul!
Lots of Love,
Jeannie

SWINGIN' AT THE SAVOY

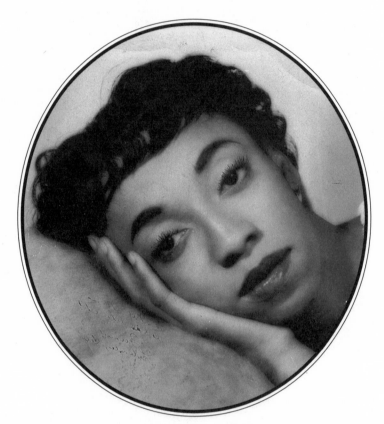

Norma Miller in Los Angeles in 1941

Swingin' at the Savoy

THE MEMOIR OF A JAZZ DANCER

Norma Miller
with Evette Jensen

TEMPLE UNIVERSITY PRESS
PHILADELPHIA

Temple University Press, Philadelphia 19122
Copyright © 1996 by Temple University
All rights reserved
Published 1996
Printed in the United States of America

∞   The paper used in this publication meets the requirements
of the American National Standard for Information Sciences—
Permanence of Paper for Printed Library Materials
ANSI Z39.48-1984

Text designed by JUDITH MARTIN WATERMAN

LIBRARY OF CONGRESS CATALOGING-IN-PUBLICATION DATA
Miller, Norma, 1919–
     Swingin' at the Savoy : the memoir of a jazz dancer /
     Norma Miller with Evette Jensen.
        p. cm.
     Includes bibliographical references.
     ISBN 1-56639-494-5 (CLOTH : alk. paper)
     1. Jazz dancing—United States—History—20th century.
2. Miller, Norma, 1919–   .   3. Women dancers—United
States—Biography.   I. Jensen, Evette.   II. Title.
GV1784.M556   1996
792.8—dc20   96-20104
                                                        CIP

This book is dedicated to
all you Swingin' dancers around the world.

▲

Remember, keep on Swingin'
Cause it don't mean a thing if it ain't got that Swing.

▼ CONTENTS

▼ ACKNOWLEDGMENTS

There are so many wonderful people who deserve special thanks for all they have given over the years. Indeed, too many to list. May you all know who you are and that you are deeply appreciated. For their help with the book, we offer our sincere thanks to the following exceptional individuals: Our agent Harriet Bernstein, and contributors Ernie Smith, Bob Crease, Bob Bailey, Jon Hendricks, and Joe Williams. To our editor, Janet Francendese, we give our gratitude for her patience and understanding. To Norma's sister, Dot, we give thanks for her special brand of compassion and generosity. And last, but certainly not least, we thank "-B-" without whose support, champagne, and sustenance we couldn't have made it. Thank you all for believing in us.

"I met Ernie, who is a jazz historian, in '84. I couldn't believe how much he knew on that he had all kinds of film and photographs. He had my whole life on film. He had things I didn't even have."

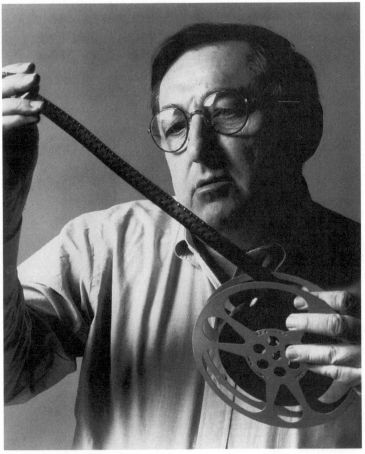

Ernie Smith, jazz historian.

Portrait of the Swing Era

A PREFACE
BY ERNIE SMITH

Conventional jazz history generally demarcates the Swing Era as a time between, roughly, 1935 and 1945. Actually, these dates reflect academic convenience more than reality when one takes into account both the music's incubation and later transitional periods. Nevertheless, the hugely successful Palomar Ballroom engagement in Los Angeles on August 21, 1935, of the still struggling Benny Goodman Orchestra is regarded as the start of a period when the public acceptance of jazz broke precedent with the past.

These years were dominated by a remarkable run of creative musicianship and its rare melding with taste. This wedding of commerce and art, if you will, was unique in many ways and left a lasting influence on mainstream American life and culture.

High art, generally speaking, is a vanguard form of expression that advances the frontiers of a culture. When significant modifications occur in the social and economic structure of society, they are almost inevitably accompanied by changes in the nature and quality, not only of high art, but also of the

popular arts. America's 1929 Wall Street stock-market crash
sent the country into a deep, long, economic slump that resulted in the Great Depression of some ten years' duration.
Popular music and jazz, which seemed to have paused in development, were actually going through an important transition. Even before 1929, popularizers in the form of arrangers,
vocalists, and dance bands were steadily moving what had been
a largely improvisational endeavor at the hands of small groups
of musicians toward the next big change.

The early, post–World War I bands, which catered to the
commercial interests of social dancers, often played easily obtainable stock arrangements and were feeding the interests of
a fast-growing, dance-obsessed public. These popular dance
bands were led by, among others, Art Hickman, Paul Specht,
The California Ramblers, Abe Lyman, Ted Lewis, Vincent
Lopez, Roger Wolfe Kahn, Jean Goldkette, and particularly,
Paul Whiteman who employed the pioneering arranging talents of Ferde Grofé and Bill Challis. The orchestras of Wilbur
Sweatman, Carroll Dickerson, Charles Elgar, Erskine Tate,
The Missourians, and Sammy Stewart had reputations in vaudeville or theater and were somewhat divorced from the dance
but cannot be discounted because of their role in shaping public
musical taste for "hot" music, thereby contributing to the
emergence of big-band jazz.

Following World War I, dance bands played to a dancing
public that continued expanding right through the Prohibition years of the Roaring Twenties. The Charleston, in all its
variations, and the Fox Trot reigned supreme. Couples were
one- and two-stepping on hundreds of dance spaces all over
the land. Punishing dance marathons regularly made news.
Records produced by a burgeoning recording industry rap-

idly spread the infection, which eventually leaped across the Atlantic. English dance bands picked up the beat, however tempered, for, say, a tea dance at the genteel Savoy or Mayfair Hotel. But it took the World War II influx of thousands of jitterbugging GIS to capture the imagination and kindle a fire under the feet of the "jiving" Britishers.

Aspiring band leaders and musicians, noting the success of these earlier orchestras, began to form dance bands whose demands for jazz-based music produced a cadre of innovative composer-player-arrangers who laid the stylistic foundation for the soon-to-emerge swing bands. Most of these talented musicians were African American, although there were a number of notable exceptions. Gene Gifford, who was the main arranger for the Casa Loma Orchestra, Joseph "Fud" Livingston, Dean Kincaide, and Isham Jones, who lead a band of his own, were some of the white talents whose arrangements were both inspiring and influential. But the more innovative, powerful ideas that furthered the development of orchestral jazz, that is, "swing," emerged from the African-American experience: Jelly Roll Morton, Duke Ellington, Don Redman, John Nesbitt, Jimmy Mundy, Edgar Sampson, Benny Carter, Eddie Durham, Mary Lou Williams, Horace Henderson, and Sy Oliver. Fletcher Henderson, who led a succession of pioneering and highly influential dance orchestras from about 1934 to 1939, was key in the creation of an environment within which it was possible for idealistic jazz musicians to play interesting, exciting, and challenging orchestrations, that were, at the same time, commercially viable. These musicians introduced, among other things, writing for specific orchestra sections—trumpets and trombones (brass), the clarinets and saxophones (reeds)—while at the same time providing opportunities for brilliant soloists to display their virtuosity. Through some very fundamental changes in the rhythm section, the stage was set for what was to come.

Certainly, by the early 1930s, the gradual replacement of the rhythmically-limiting tuba and staccato-sounding banjo with the plucked, upright bass and the more melodic, softer strum of the guitar resulted in a major change from the jerky, stop-time rhythms of the Charleston era. Most importantly, beat-keeping by the drummer went to the more shimmering, flowing, sound of the ride cymbal, the high hat, and the continuous whisk of wire brushes across the snare drum. Thus, with each of the four beats getting equal emphasis (4/4 time), the rhythm became more fluid and constant. There were other changes, of course, but these were most crucial to the pulse that drove swing bands. To this mix can be added the arrangers' new approaches, such as the call-and-response patterns embodied in the riffing passages of one section against another—brass against reeds and so forth—with star soloist improvisations soaring over these same riff figures. Additional touches like crescendos ending in brass smears followed by sudden orchestral breaks with only the rhythm section audible, the unison saxophone passages, the breaks; all went into creating music that made the impulse to dance virtually irresistible. The best of the Lindy Hoppers, sensitive to these devices, used steps and dance patterns that not only reflected the music, but also provided counterpoint. Thus, the lead in a Lindy partnership had to act as choreographer. This made it important to understand the band's style and be familiar with its arrangements. An aspiring Lindy dancer who is insensitive to these swing band tenets, is doomed to a rather mechanical, though acceptable, version of the dance. A good understanding of what big-band swing is about on the other hand, can result in a most satisfying experience on the dance floor without the need to resort to air steps. This later addition to the Lindy gave the Savoy Ballroom dancers, like Whitey's Lindy Hoppers, a decided edge in competitions such as New York City's annual Harvest Moon Ball. Add to this the sheer exhilaration of moving with a swing-sympathetic and sensitive partner, opportunities for injecting humor and whimsy, a chance to "get down in the alley" when the mood is right and to insert personal improvisational steps and touches, and you have Lindy dancing at its best.

"Big band" and "dance band" were terms used to describe Swing Era orchestras, which, generally, had swelled to a standard fourteen or sixteen pieces by this time. Their music could range from the sweet genteel bounce of a society band to the uncomplicated, but driving, blues-oriented swing of the Count Basie Band. While most of these bands catered to the whole of the dancing community, the distinction between them was based on the segment to which their music appealed. Dance bands such as Irving Aaronson's, Jan Garber's, Eddie Duchin's, Meyer Davis's, Sammy Kay's, Freddie Martin's, or Guy Lombardo's (when Lombardo played the Savoy Ballroom, strangely enough, he established an attendance record), were very successful with the conservative social dancer because they offered a dependable but unchallenging beat. These dancers are best described as favoring a style that leaned heavily on the Irene and Vernon Castle school, on English ballroom dancing, and on other European standards of social dance.

At the other end of the spectrum were the hard swinging organizations of Count Basie, Lucky Millinder, Benny Goodman, Andy Kirk, Chick Webb (the long time Savoy house band), Jimmie Lunceford, Erskine Hawkins, Horace Henderson, Jay McShann, among others, whose pushing-the-beat music not only generated the heat and challenge so necessary for inspired Lindy dancing but also hastened the departure of some accepted norms of dance etiquette.

In between were bands of every stripe that produced very acceptable, sometimes even exciting, dance music that appealed to most dancers including the Lindy Hoppers—Glenn Miller, Gene Krupa, Larry Clinton, Glen Gray, Jimmy and Tommy Dorsey, Harry James, Artie Shaw, Noble Sissle, Jan Savitt (whose shuffle rhythm seemed to appeal to the Shag dancer), and Bob Crosby. They played a balance of ballads and novelty vocals along with memorable swing instrumentals. Oddly enough, the music of Duke Ellington, one of the giants and seminal figures in jazz and American music, created problematic music for the better Lindy dancers. When he chose to appeal directly to them, Ellington could produce a swinging "C-Jam Blues," "In a Mellotone," or "Take the A Train." But many of his exciting compositions were filled with strange and interesting harmonies, surprising juxtapositions, and shifting rhythms and were sprinkled throughout with dissonances. These made some of Ellington's greatest works unacceptable pieces for the avid Lindy Hopper. Duke's resistance to being categorized as just a swing band often cost him the admiration of the best of the Lindy Hoppers.

Many earlier dance bands relied on easily obtainable stock arrangements with alterations here and there to add interest. In order to inject hot or peppy touches, leaders employed individual musicians with established reputations as good, jazz-driven, improvisatory players who were expected to raise the jazz standard of many bands to dancer's expectations. This form of dance music was played in a variety of venues such as speakeasies, cabarets, hotels, restaurants, and later, along the ballroom circuit or in nightclub dance casinos. What was accepted as a form of pure jazz was still largely perceived as African American in origin, but black musicians, with some exceptions, rarely had the opportunity to play directly for downtown whites. Those white folks with a developed taste for hot music or some other aspect of black culture, made frequent visits uptown, to experience the real thing on home ground. Black urban enclaves such as Chicago's South Side; the Central Avenue district in Los Angeles; Kansas City, St. Louis, Omaha, Atlanta, and, particularly, New York's Harlem, were but a few that served as magnets for the culturally curious.

Harlem's Cotton Club and Small's Paradise, the Grand Terrace in Chicago, and Sebastian's Cotton Club in the Los Angeles area drew a steady stream of white patronage. The Savoy was the first ballroom to integrate. These inquisitive whites included, among others, hot music devotees, musicians looking for fresh ideas, songwriters seeking inspiration, artists and literati, dancers who wanted to be on the cutting edge, show business folk, thinking liberals and intellectuals, people seeking new entertainments, and slumming thrill seekers. All were acting (unconsciously or consciously) as a kind of pollinator. For whatever purpose, they would introduce what they heard uptown into their own downtown environments. This cross-fertilization reached a crescendo in the years between the 1920s and mid-'30s, a period of fecundity in African-American culture known as the Harlem Renaissance. A cynical observation by many Harlem residents at the time was that "Harlem was ours during the day but belonged to white folks at night."

Although black bands, such as those led by Fletcher Henderson, had played for white dancers at New York's Roseland Ballroom in 1924, with the young, trumpet playing jazz genius Louis Armstrong in the brass section, there was still a considerable cultural gap between uptown and downtown. Not so much within the groups with specific musical tastes but between African-American culture and that of the downtown mass public. Mainstream Americans still regarded uptown as a mysterious sub-culture filled with a people and imagery reflective of the years of slavery and the minstrel era. It often took time for the evolving and innovative ideas in art, music, and dance within the black community to seep out into the American mainstream. Marshall Stearns defined this time gap, or crossover period, as a kind of cultural lag. The rapid development of the phonograph, recordings, radio, and motion pictures lessened the time it took for the cross-fertilization process to show its impact on white culture. As long as the two cultures remained so separate more pollinators, both white and black, were needed.

The enthusiastic and perceptive jazz gadabout and strong civil-rights advocate, John Hammond, was one such influential pollinator. He worked tirelessly to bring uptown musical development, its innovators and practitioners, and black social concerns, to the attention of downtown sensibilities. There were others of course, Carl Van Vechten, Stanley Dance, Helen Oakley, and Marshall Stearns, but Hammond was particularly enthusiastic about black jazz. Through his well-developed network and connections within the recording industry and the press, with both black and white entrepreneurial booking agents, band leaders, and club owners he was able to translate his enthusiasm into positive action. In addition, the pioneering output of so many uptown bands such as Fletcher Henderson's, Don Redman's, and Duke Ellington's, to mention only three, resulted in a gradual and inexorable success of swing music. As a result, jazz and social dancing, both solidly linked, would swing hand-in-hand into the Swing Era. The Black Bottom, the Charleston, the many animal dances like the Bunny Hug, Grizzly Bear, and Turkey Trot, were either giving way or being absorbed piecemeal by the gradual development of a new uptown dance that reflected the fresh spirit of swing and suited the music perfectly. That dance was the Savoy-created Lindy Hop.

Americans experienced dance crazes with some regularity through the Ragtime years and the Jazz Age, but nothing quite compared to what happened during the Swing Era. Social dancing became serious business indeed. An entire generation took to the Harlem-born, Savoy-style Lindy Hop (or Jitterbug) and later, the Big Apple, Truckin', Peckin', the Boogie Woogie, the Suzi-Q, the Shag, and the Shim Sham, although some of these dances and steps had their roots in earlier generations of dance from other regions of the country. The heavily blues-oriented music played in hundreds of juke joints and honky tonks in the South and Southwest profoundly affected dance steps and styles that came North with migrating blacks who were seeking more hospitable surroundings and greater economic opportunity.

Additional cross-fertilization was evident in the rise of Western Swing in the early 1930s, a music that drew upon country, popular, and jazz. Stressing a strong beat with jazz-like improvisations on the steel guitar and bowed fiddle, it was heard in dance halls along the Gulf Coast and throughout the Southwest, particularly in Oklahoma and Texas, and eventually, as far east as Kentucky. Ideal for dancing, a lively mixture of traditional country square dancing, ballroom, the Fox Trot, and, in later years, the addition of the Lindy Hop–like moves and patterns, it was immensely popular with regional dancers.

One can only speculate as to how profound an effect this sort of cultural cross-fertilization had on American social dance. But without a doubt, whatever the mix, it was pronounced and original. A popular dance comes into being as the result of a long, complex process, and, because it is vernacular, as in the case of the Lindy Hop, its finite origins can be virtually impossible to trace. There was mention of the Texas Tommy, along with other dances, that the older musicians described as having some similarities to the Lindy Hop. But this much we can be positive about, Swing music spurred its development, and the best place to hear that music and see the dance performed was in Harlem at the Savoy Ballroom, which opened for business on March 12, 1926, while the Charleston era was winding down.

The beginnings of the Lindy Hop can be seen in *After Seben*, a ten minute short subject filmed in 1928 and released by Paramount in 1929. It starred the minstrel show–trained dancer James Barton, who, in kinky wig and blackface, introduced three pairs of champion dancers recruited from the Savoy Ballroom. They were among the Savoy dancing elite whose acknowledged "King," George "Shorty" Snowden, was one of the dancers. They appeared in a sequence staged as a dance competition with Snowden and his partner dancing last. Snowden was extraordinarily riveting as they danced to a hot rendition of "Sweet Sue," played by Chick Webb and his orchestra. Although these seminal dancers used steps associated with the now-departing Charleston and the even earlier

Cakewalk, they also employed some new but well-developed and recognizable steps, including the swing-out or breakaway, a key dance maneuver that was to become the cornerstone step of the Lindy Hop. Snowden was not only a sensational dancer but an inventive one, and a number of steps are attributed to him, one bearing his name—the "Shorty George"—which Count Basie immortalized with a 1938 recording.

As the Lindy developed, the best of the Savoy Lindy Hoppers, who favored the original floor version, seemed to be in constant motion with steps strung together into connected patterns that produced a non-stop, but beautifully controlled, and often, superbly elegant, partner dance. One remained loose and flexible from the hips down. It was not until Benny Goodman's ascendancy to the King of Swing that white mainstream kids adopted the dance en masse (the cultural lag again). These kids tended to emphasize strength with more hopping, verticality, bounce, and arm pumping, rather than the smooth, horizontal flow of the uptown original. The term Jitterbug came into use to describe these dancers, a combination word that had a black origin, often with meanings other than dance, for instance, Jitter Sauce, meaning liquor, and Jitter Bug, one who likes to drink liquor. In 1934 Cab Calloway wrote a tune called "Jitter Bug," which predates the white Lindy explosion in 1936. Jitterbug became synonymous with Lindy Hop, and the two terms were used interchangeably. Then, to later dancers and dance historians, the Jitterbug and its parent the Lindy Hop, although virtually identical in basic execution, again became two distinctly different dances as the Jitterbug came to be defined by its verticality, its hopping up and down. It brings to mind Jimmie Lunceford's 1939 hit recording "'Taint What You Do (It's the Way That 'Cha Do It)." This writer learned to dance the Lindy in Pittsburgh where the term Lindy Hop was rarely, if ever, used. When seeking a suitable partner at any ballroom, one generally asked, "Do you Jitterbug?" or "Do you fast dance?" A dance evening would generally include a "Jitterbug Special."

Gunther Schuller offers a crucial insight into Lindy dancing. Although apologetic for the lack of real expertise in the subject, he nevertheless possesses, not only a good ear for swing but a sharp eye as well when he notes.

> It is my impression from viewing films of dancers in the Swing Era that in fast numbers, white dancers were much more vertical in their movements, vigorously bobbing up and down, while black dancers were much more horizontal and wide-ranging. This verticality and stiffness had its exact corollary in the drumming of most white drummers, until the likes of Dave Tough and Buddy Rich came along.[1]

To this, I can only add—Amen!

As both swing music and the Lindy Hop's popularity soared, ballrooms, both large and small, opened everywhere across the land and, like movie palaces, the architecture and interiors often had exotic influences. Spanish-Moorish touches, red velvet or gilt borrowed from Europe's French and Italian palaces, and ceilings with moving clouds and twinkling stars turned some of these recreational spaces into dance-floored marvels of baroque splendor. A patron could be transported into a wonderful world that combined exciting music with a fantasy environment. Major urban centers possessed more than one such dance palace, but even small towns could boast of a dance hall. They sprang up on oceanfront boardwalks, in metro-

[1] Schuller, Gunther, *The Swing Era* (New York: Oxford University Press, 1989), 241n.

politan suburbs, or in popular amusement parks. Lavish, elegant, ballrooms such as Harlem's block-long Savoy, Roseland in New York's Times Square area, or the Aragon and Trianon in Chicago, not to mention the Palomar and Palladium in Los Angeles, packed in hundreds and thousands of dancers nightly. And everywhere, the Savoy Lindy Hop, or some altered version of it reigned supreme. Some ballrooms, like the Savoy, offered two bands so the music never stopped. As further appeasement to the enormous public appetite for a social evening, most nightclubs would provide a small postage-sized dance floor, ringed with tables and seating, offering a swing-trio, quartet, or other combination, but at the very least, a juke box, to provide the necessary music. Frank Dailey's Meadowbrook in Cedar Grove, New Jersey, and the Glen Island Casino in New Rochelle, New York, showcased big-name bands for their dancing patronage. With the automobile as a cheap, well-established means of getting about, traveling to out-of-town spots, called roadhouses, became common. These places provided food and drink and a dance floor with some sort of swing music, either live or recorded, and became popular after-hours extensions for those wishing to dance beyond the closing time of regular ballrooms. Regional dance bands and swing aggregations, popular with the local dance population, flourished and were enough in demand to provide comfortable livings for hometown musicians, who either by choice or chance, did not make it on to the national dance-band circuit. Dancing to recordings at school gymnasiums, church meeting rooms, lodges, YMCAs, social clubs, bar-and-grills of every variety, and one's own home were alternatives to the formality and expense of big ballrooms. Dancers, whether Lindy or otherwise, were not great

consumers of liquor because drinking could seriously interfere with one's ability to execute moves and steps. Therefore,
soft drinks became popular thirst quenchers.

What were the effects of the Swing Era on mainstream
culture? Fashion and dress might be a place to begin. With
the youthful fan, or Jitterbug, what one wore loudly spoke to
the preoccupation with the world of swing. Some attire was
reflective of musicians or band vocalists because much of the
era's young people were ardent about the energetic dances
the music spawned. As the number-one dance, the Lindy Hop,
described as choreographed swing music, had its own dress
codes. The rolled stockings of the Roaring Twenties flapper
gave way to Swing Era bobby socks, saddle shoes, sweaters,
and skirts, which were flared at the bottom to permit vigor-
ous execution of Lindy steps. When women wished to appear
more dressy, a one or two-piece dress, blouse, hosiery, and
ankle-strap, medium heeled shoes were the vogue. Males,
much more the peacocks, often borrowed from the dress styles
of musicians, sporting pleated, pegged trousers, wide at the
knees and narrow at the cuffs, a key chain looped from belt to
pocket, and a double-breasted suit jacket of a one-button roll
style with wide, padded shoulders. This tailoring referred to
the suit-jacket lapel that was pressed into a long, soft roll that
closed low at the waist with a single button: "the reat pleat
with a drape shape." Cardigan sport jackets were also popular,
with evenly spaced, vertical striped neckties, which could be,
with studied casualness, carelessly left to dangle outside of
one's jacket to establish Swing Era nonchalance. Pork-pie hats
à la Lester Young, Coleman Hawkins, Gene Krupa, Duke
Ellington, Roy Eldridge, and scores of swing musicians, became the chapeau of choice. The flashy, outrageous zoot suit,

a Harlem-favored extreme popularized by such charismatic figures as band leader-vocalist Cab Calloway, was worn by a small number of devotees and lasted into the 1950s where post-swing hipsters and the Latinos of Los Angeles took up the style as their fashion statement. A candidate for the quintessential icon of the era is the male hepcat—decked out in full-dress swing attire, a zoot suit topped off with a wide-brimmed hat, standing with knees slightly bent, shoulders a bit hunched, arms at the side with his index fingers pointing down along the seams of his trousers to sharp-toed, wing-tipped, brown and white Florsheim shoes, and looking enigmatically detached, content, and "sent."

One could usually distinguish, by attire, between the collegiate, the urban dweller, the well-to-do, and the rest of the Lindy crowd. College campus swingers and eastern Shag dancers favored the bobby-sox, saddle-shoe, clean-cut look, while the urban hepcat went for the sophisticated, sharp look. These styles changed a great deal with America's entry into World War II. In order to conserve precious fabric needed for uniforms, parachutes, and other wartime use, tailoring eliminated not only pleats and generous knee room for trousers, but cuffs as well. Shoulder padding and jacket lengths also suffered. Ladies' nylon hose were replaced with tan leg paints. Wartime measures affected everything, from shellac for records to gasoline for automobiles. Big bands lost men to the draft and the rapidly expanding armed forces.

If the garment industry profited by tailoring apparel to Swing Era fashion, Hollywood also knew a good thing when it heard it. The studios hoped to hear cash-register jingle through exploitation of this new musical craze. Swing became big box office. Hollywood produced over fifty films with "swing" in the title, testimony to the drawing power of the era's pied piper. Movies were soon serving up every aspect of the Swing Era in dozens of films. Large swing orchestras and small combos, vocalists and vocal groups, star soloists, swing characters spouting swing argot, or "jive," were written into all sorts of screenplays for feature films, short subjects, and even cartoons. Benny Goodman's Orchestra appeared in Paramount's *The Big Broadcast of 1937* and in Warner Brothers 1937 *Hollywood Hotel*, which also spotlighted the original, racially mixed Benny Goodman Quartet with Teddy Wilson, Gene Krupa, and Lionel Hampton. Louis Armstrong, Duke Ellington, Les Hite, Harry James, both Dorsey orchestras, Ella Fitzgerald, Peggy Lee, Fats Waller, and others, appeared in film after film in cameo appearances. Some had dialogue and honest-to-goodness acting roles. As the era gained momentum Hollywood cranked out dozens and dozens of ten- and fifteen-minute short subjects completely given over to one swing aggregation after another, from the Jimmie Lunceford and Gene Krupa orchestras, to Al Cooper and his Savoy Sultans, or the Mills Brothers.

The dancers were drawn from Whitey's Lindy Hoppers, a performance group of amateur but superior, Savoy dancers, organized and nurtured by a perceptive and entrepreneurial Herbert White—a sometime bouncer at the ballroom, who also knew a good thing when he saw it and shaped these dancers into a highly skilled, professional unit. Their initial movie appearance was in the 1937 MGM Marx Brothers' *A Day at the Races* with Duke Ellington's great vocalist Ivie Anderson singing "All God's Children Got Rhythm." These remarkable young dancers provided the film its production number with two or three minutes of spectacular Lindy virtuosity that still manages to astonish and inspire present day dancers. Current groups such as Sweden's "Rhythm Hotshots" and England's "Jiving Lindy Hoppers" looked to this extraordinary footage not only for inspiration, but also as instruction for their own re-creations. A different mix of Whitey's dancers appeared in the 1944 film *Hellzapoppin'* featuring the zany antics of the comic team Olsen and Johnson. This performance took the aerial-step Lindy to new heights, achieving a kind of Lindy Hop summit that remains unequaled to this day.

By 1940 public high-traffic areas such as amusement arcades, neighborhood bars, taverns, restaurants, bus and train stations, hotel lobbies, and the like, could boast the installation of a new audio-visual device called Panoram, which offered both music and entertainment. This video jukebox wedded two technologies: the ever popular jukebox and movies. By mounting a sixteen millimeter motion-picture projector inside, these coin-operated machines offered three-minute films, called soundies, on large screens, which enabled the viewer to both see and hear the artist of choice. Many of the Swing Era's most popular and important artists appeared in either straight performance or mini-dramatizations of recording hits. Duke Ellington, Gene Krupa, Fats Waller, Cab Calloway, dancer Bill Robinson, vocalists Anita O'Day, Mel Torme, and Whitey's Lindy Hoppers, along with a horde of lesser-known talents, appeared in these minimovies. Adding this film library to the enormous output of the record companies and the daily radio broadcasts (called remotes) from important music and dance locations, provided Americans with a cornucopia of swing material to satisfy not only every taste, but also to keep the swing juggernaut in high gear.

Broadway took up the beat with *The Hot Mikado* (1939, originally called *The Swing Mikado*); the short-lived *Swingin' the Dream* (1939), which showcased Whitey's dancers; Ellington's *Jump for Joy* (1941), which opened and closed in Los Angeles; and the musical revue *The Seven Lively Arts* (1944), which featured a Benny Goodman all-star group in a specialty spot.

Pioneering disc jockeys such as Al Jarvis and Martin Block, both claiming credit for originating radio's *Make Believe Ballroom*, along with others, were also key to the promotion of swing bands. The *Fitch Bandwagon* and *Coca Cola's Spotlight Bands* were but two, out of many, sponsored radio shows that helped popularize swing.

Music publications like *Downbeat, Metronome, Tempo, Band Leaders*, and occasionally, *Esquire* were but a few of the magazines that devoted themselves to the swing scene. Song sheets that printed lyrics to most of the Tin Pan Alley hits came out periodically. *Downbeat* inaugurated its annual reader's poll to select fandom's favorite swing artists, while *Metronome* magazine, through a poll of its own, selected musicians for a *Metronome* All-Star Band recording. An imposing body of jazz critics and writers, many who are still with us, came to the fore during this period—reviewing records, concerts, ballroom and nightclub appearances, stage shows that headlined swing talent and keeping the readership aware of what was going on in the world of swing. Important books and articles about the rise of jazz and swing were written during this period. Fans got together and formed hot clubs. Rare record collecting and discographical research became a productive obsession for a dedicated few.

Art and writing reflected the trend. Although not great literature, novels and fiction drew on the swing life for inspiration. *Jazz Band* by Wyatt Randel, Richard English's *Strictly Ding Dong and Other Swing Stories*, and Dale Curran's *Piano in the Band* with a foreword by Benny Goodman, were a few.[2]

Painters from the world of fine art also found inspiration in the swing scene. The cubist-influenced American, Stuart Davis painted *Swing Landscape* (1938) and *The Mellow Pad* (1945–1951). Both paintings succeeded in making swing visible through the use of hard-edged shapes and bright, crisp color. Piet Mondrian, an emigrant Dutch painter (he and Davis were fellow jazz buffs) reached for the walking-bass figures of Boogie-Woogie, a piano blues style that resurfaced during the Swing Era, when he painted *Broadway Boogie Woogie* (1942–1943) and *Victory Boogie Woogie* (1943–1944). African-American artist Romare Bearden, with a life-long interest in jazz and the blues, painted *At the Savoy* (1974) and a number of works evocative of urban jazz and syncopation in his *4/4 Time* and *Of the Blues* series. New Orleans born Richmond Barthé, another African American, produced a beautifully expressive bronze sculpture *Lindy Hop* (1939) which celebrated the quintessential couple dance of the 1930s and '40s.

Although it did not necessarily begin with the Swing Era, the use of a specialized slang became popular and quickly found its way into everyday language. Originating largely within black communities, or with jazz musicians and the swing milieu in general, its use became essential in establishing oneself as part of the cognoscenti. Both Harlem's Dan Burley and Cab

[2] Randel, Wyatt, *Jazz Band* (New York: Greenburg, 1935); English, Richard, *Strictly Ding Dong and Other Swing Stories* (New York: Doubleday, Doran & Co., 1938); and Curran, Dale, *Piano in the Band* (New York: Reynal & Hitchcock, 1940).

Calloway wrote handbooks that served as guides for the proper use of swing language such as hep (later hip), jive, cat, square, bread (money), chops, solid, blow your top, rugcutter (a swing dancer), riff, killer-diller (an all-stops-out, up-tempo arrangement), and Alligator (sometimes shortened to Gator). The lyrics to Cab Calloway's "The Jumpin' Jive" (1939) was a classic example of the use of swing slang.

Concert halls, first successfully invaded in the 1920s by dance bands led by Vincent Lopez and Paul Whiteman, now saw one swing concert after another fill the seats of these bastions of high culture with excited, cheering, foot-stomping, dancing-in-the-aisles, swing fans. Again, Benny Goodman led the way with his famed 1938 Carnegie Hall Concert. Carnegie Hall also became the stage for two Spirituals to Swing concerts produced by the indefatigable John Hammond in 1938 and 1939, as well as a series of Duke Ellington concerts beginning in 1943. As a Judy Garland vocal in MGM's *Thousands Cheer* (1943) would enthusiastically note, "the joint is really jumpin' in Carnegie Hall."

The Great Depression, during which approximately one-third of Americans were unemployed, was also coincidental with some of the most important years of the Swing Era. Times were difficult. Big Bands and the popularity of social dancing and the Lindy Hop, along with the movies, provided both inexpensive and supremely satisfying recreative social activity for the masses. Swing music and related entertainments played a key role in creating hope and diversion for a population experiencing chronic unemployment, economic despair, and a future full of uncertainties.

Franklin Roosevelt, elected to the presidency in 1933 on a platform that promised Americans a "New Deal," carried the burden of recovery with a long list of let's-try-it ideas. Some were effective, others were not, but the movement always seemed forward and fostered renewed optimism about the future. By 1939, two world's fairs, New York's "World of Tomorrow" and San Francisco's "Golden Gate International Exposition," seemed to signal the dawn of better times. With an impossibly grueling performance schedule, Whitey's Lindy Hoppers were a six-month attraction at the New York fair.

The Swing Era witnessed significant economic and social change, not only for white Americans but for African Americans and other minorities as well. Considerable groundwork had been laid by earlier individuals and organizations such as Marcus Garvey, W.E.B. DuBois, and the Niagara Movement, The National Association for the Advancement of Colored People (NAACP), The National Urban League, and others, whose social agendas included civil and voting rights, greater educational and economic opportunity, social equality, and an end to lynching, to name just a few. Black writers, artists, and intellectuals associated with the Harlem Renaissance concerned themselves with validating "The New Negro" and establishing a sense of racial pride.

Sports figures such as Jesse Owens, the track and field gold medalist of the Berlin Olympics in 1936; Joe Louis, son of an Alabama sharecropper and world heavyweight champion from 1937 to 1949, who exuded decency and a quiet strength that was an inspiration to all; and Satchel Paige, black baseball great, who was among the first to break the color barrier in that sport, were all exemplary role models, not only in the black community, but throughout the world as well.

In Washington, D.C., in 1939, when denied access to Constitutional Hall for a concert, Marian Anderson, one of the world's great contraltos, with the help of Eleanor Roosevelt, struck a blow for equality and justice when she sang on the steps of the Lincoln Memorial instead.

Without the benefit of a formal platform or publicly stated policy, a number of individuals intimately involved with the Swing Era helped liberalize a highly segregated music and entertainment industry. Their efforts succeeded, albeit modestly, in gaining higher visibility for blacks in these areas. John Hammond, who had the ear of Benny Goodman, advised him to hire the best swing musicians he could find. Thus, he hired pianist Teddy Wilson and vibraphonist Lionel Hampton, and along with himself and Gene Krupa on drums, formed the first Benny Goodman Quartet in 1936. Later he would feature other black musicians, like the legendary guitarist Charlie Christian; Ellington's great trumpet star, Cootie Williams; and bassist Slam Stewart. Racially mixed groups and bands had real problems when tours took them West or through the South. In the North, segregationist attitudes took a more subtle form but were just as oppressive. Accommodations, food, and lodging for blacks was of particular concern everywhere when swing bands went on the road. When band leader Charlie Barnet took on a just-starting-out Lena Horne as his vocalist, he resorted to subterfuge at hotel check-in counters, presenting her as a Cuban singer while other band members spoke Spanish-sounding gibberish to convince a skeptical clerk. Artie Shaw briefly employed Billie Holiday as his band vocalist. Over the swing years, Charlie Barnet hired, among others, black trumpeters Peanuts Holland, Sidney DeParis, Charlie Shavers, Dick Vance, Clark Terry, and Al Killian, as well as trombonist Trummy Young, bassist Oscar Pettiford, and pianist Ram Ramirez. Tommy Dorsey had also hired Charlie Shavers in 1945 to play in his trumpet section and to occasionally sing. These swing band leaders stated that the hiring of black musicians was not done out of any conviction to make a social statement but rather because they wanted the best talents available. Some musicians, like Roy Eldridge, a leading trumpet player at the time, joined the Gene Krupa Orchestra in 1941 and, later, Artie Shaw's, as well. Segregation and bigotry left him with bitter memories of both experiences. Nevertheless, some real progress was being made in presenting racially-mixed orchestras and entertainments.

Ballroom floors were not the only places where the influence of swing was evident. The theatrical stage, where tap dancing, whose roots go back to well before the minstrel period, had experienced a tremendous boost from the syncopations of the ragtime era. Subsequently, jazz and swing played a particularly significant role in elevating the percussions of rhythm tap to the level of an art form. Tent shows, vaudeville, revues, Broadway shows, night clubs, and sound movies provided entertainments in which tap could flourish. Big bands, in addition to providing social dance music, also became major stage attractions. Comics, vocalists, and dancers were added to their appearances in order to round out an entertainment package. These swing band–centered units toured the theater circuits, offering a two-hour stage show in addition to a first-run movie. Groups from Whitey's Lindy Hoppers traveled with such packages as did many of the country's greatest tappers.

Bunny Briggs, one of the most innovative and original tap talents, whose seemingly carefree performances were crammed with wit, dramatic explosions, and fluid elegance, danced with the orchestras of Count Basie, Earl Hines, and particularly

Charlie Barnet. The astonishing Condos Brothers toured with Basie, Ellington, Lunceford, the Dorseys, and Benny Goodman. Steve Condos observed that while the melody always could be heard in their music, it also always had a swing touch. So as to be assured of getting the kind of music needed, they hired Jimmy Mundy, the talent behind so many swing band blockbusters, to create arrangements for them. Many of the legendary tap dancers came to be associated with particular swing bands. Baby Lawrence with Count Basie; Teddy Hale with Louis Jordan; Jimmy Slyde with Duke Ellington and Basie; Bunny Briggs with Charlie Barnet; Ralph Brown and Honi Coles with Cab Calloway. Peg Leg Bates danced with virtually every important swing band—Charlie Barnet, Cab Calloway, Claude Hopkins, Jimmie Lunceford, and Count Basie. The Count Basie Orchestra was particularly admired by, not only the tappers, but the Savoy Lindy Hoppers as well. Basie, in turn, loved and respected dancers—whether social or theatrical. He rarely toured the theater circuit without a dancer or two. A number of his original compositions gave tribute to them, his "Baby Lawrence" and "Honi Coles" are but two examples.

The Japanese attack at Pearl Harbor on December 7, 1941, catapulted America into World War II, which had been raging in Europe since 1939. Big band personnel suffered major losses to both patriotic volunteerism and selective service. Whitey's Lindy Hoppers felt the effects of the draft as well when they lost some of their most important dancing talents. Swing bands became important in boosting and maintaining morale, not only on the home front, but in the armed forces as well. Most army, navy, and air force bases could boast a resident swing orchestra, often filled with veteran players from big-name bands. These base swing groups played for on-post dances and other entertainments. Despite wartime restrictions, like curfews and shortages of gasoline and rubber for tires, which put a crimp into touring and traveling, America experienced a surprising boom in entertainment of all kinds. Show business, along with big bands, swung into high gear to meet the growing need for social diversion from the harrowing demands of fighting a major war. Big bands joined movie stars and other entertainment personalities in playing a key role in fund-raising during war bond rallies. Some of the band leaders who joined the armed forces included Artie Shaw, Claude Thornhill, Rudy Vallee, Eddie Duchin, and Ray Anthony. Veteran swing musicians such as the highly-influential tenorist Lester Young and Basie drummer Jo Jones were also called up but their experience in the service of their country was bitter indeed.

The most high-profile leader to enlist was Glenn Miller, who, with the rank of captain, formed a precedent-breaking air force band that included seasoned swing-era musicians such as Ray McKinley, Trigger Alpert, Carmen Mastren, Mel Powell, and Bernie Privin, to mention a few. The band became justly famous for playing march arrangements of "St. Louis Blues" and "Blues in the Night," which had a real sense of swing to them, a touch that often drew critical fire from old-line bandmasters and army officers alike.

Twelve-inch, unbreakable records, called V-Discs (V for Victory) produced by the Music Branch of the Army Special Services, were specifically targeted at the recreational needs of service men and women all over the world. The V-Disc catalog supplied selections that appealed to a broad-spectrum of musical taste: symphonic and classical; vocals—operatic, ballad, or novelty, along with jazz and swing. Much of it was played over the Armed Forces Radio Network. Through these special recordings, swing bands such as those of Artie Shaw, Erskine Hawkins, Duke Ellington, Harry James, Benny Goodman, Lucky Millinder, and Don Redman proved to be real morale boosters. American GIs, raised and nurtured in the swing-saturated environment of this period, spread the gospel of swing music and related dances, particularly the Lindy Hop, wherever they set foot. Newsreel footage of jitterbugging soldiers at overseas locations, at USO centers, in remote battlefield settings, at victory celebrations in the streets of Paris and London, were commonplace.

With the German surrender on May 7, 1945, and Japan's capitulation on August 14, 1945, the war years came to a close. Life back home, already considerably changed, saw the return of millions of service men and women, which would have a further impact on a changing America. A new form of jazz was in ascendance. It was called BeBop. Primarily a listener's music, it was not very dancer friendly. Big bands would make a last ditch stand over the next few years and a few, like Harry James's, Woody Herman's, Count Basie's, and Glenn Miller's (fronted by leaders other than Miller, who was a World War II missing-in-action casualty), hung on indefinitely. But for all intents and purposes, the Swing Era was over.

Norma Miller's memoir takes you step-by-step through the glorious Lindy Hop years of the Swing Era. She was there during the initial years; saw it develop, thrive, and take to the air; travel downtown, across the country, and around the globe. As part of that seminal and highly influential group, Whitey's Lindy Hoppers, she, along with dancers like Frankie

Manning (who created the first aerial step) took the dance into the movies, onto Broadway, and to London, Paris, Australia, and Brazil. Norma loves swing and the Lindy, and her story confirms their romance time and again. Her recollections illuminate one of the great periods in music, cultural history, and American dance.

Ernie Smith
New York City

Entwined in the pages of notes and interviews, with their bent corners and tattered edges, was a wonderful story. . . .

The writing of *Swingin' at the Savoy* has been an incredible experience. During our many hours of meetings, Norma made the challenging task a joy, and in the process she has become a very dear part of my family. Here in the middle of the desert, I found a gem—her name is Norma Miller. By sharing her story, her friendship, and her zest for life, Norma has given me a great gift, and I love her for it.

Evette Jensen
Las Vegas

Swingin' at the Savoy

Coming Home

I had been driving cross-country for two weeks with my two poodles and my cat, Coco. They were great traveling companions, never whining or complaining. When I decided to go home I knew that I had to drive, and I had to bring my precious pets. They were like my own children, and I could not possibly leave them in the care of anyone else. I saw the sign that read "Lincoln Tunnel" and knew that at last I was nearing New York. Finally, home.

When I decided to return to New York I called my sister, Dot. Good ol' Dot, I could always depend on her, she was the mediator between my Mama and me. As I headed toward the tunnel I could just imagine how their telephone conversation had gone.

"Hello Mama, I just got a call from Bunny, she wants to come home."

"Well, what's stopping her? Tell her to get her ass home."

"She needs money."

"So, she needs money. Don't she have any?"

"I guess not, she's asking us to send her the money so she can come home."

"She needs money. Are you crazy? She's been gone all this time and still don't have a pot to piss in. What she needs is a husband!"

"She's bringing her poodles with her."

"Poodles? I always thought she was crazy."

"She's bringing her cat too."

"Now I know she's crazy! I'll be damned. Well, send it to her. I guess I'm a little crazy too."

Countless memories filled my head. As I exited at 41st Street, I turned left automatically as I had done so many times in the past traveling between New York and New Jersey. Turning uptown onto 8th Avenue, my mind drifted when suddenly, a taxi driver brought me back to reality. He cut me off in typical New York fashion yelling, "Hey you dumb bitch! Where in the hell did you learn to drive?" I was shocked for a moment, and then realizing where I was, I began to laugh. "Welcome to New York." Yes, I knew I was home at last.

It didn't take long to get back in the swing of things. I drove toward the park and entered at 59th Street, nearing Harlem, my old stomping grounds. As I emerged at 110th Street I saw that Harlem had changed. Lenox Avenue was now called Adam Clayton Powell. The further up I drove, the more change I saw. Approaching 140th Street, where the Savoy had been was the Delano Apartments; what was once the grand Savoy entrance was now a Woolworth's. I parked and got out of my car, overwhelmed.

It seemed that my whole past had been eliminated—all the great happenings, the big bands, the great singers, the dancing. The Lindy Hop had been created there! But now it was hard to believe they had existed at all, but they had existed, and I was living proof.

It felt as if the memories had been wiped out deliberately and would not exist for future generations.

We had danced at the Savoy. We created America's only dance and took it around the world, that was what the Savoy represented. People everywhere are dancing that dance today, and it is because of what we created there. All of the memories of that time in Harlem, our entire history, was erased.

Standing there, I could almost hear my mother's voice calling me to come in from the fire escape, and I could almost pick up the scent of frying onions and pork chops.

As children, we lived in an apartment behind the Savoy with our mother, and on hot summer nights the windows of the ballroom were open. Every night when the music would start my sister Dot and I would take up a seat on the fire escape. The music flowed from the windows. The air was hot and as sticky as warm molasses, but we would sit and watch and listen as though we were sitting in a theater's box seats.

"I told you kids to come in from the fire escape, it's time you were in bed."

"Oh Ma, just a few more minutes, I want to hear the end of this song."

"Don't 'Oh Ma' me, I said come in and I mean come in now! That damned music, keeping a person awake all night. . . ."

Mama was still complaining as we rushed off to bed.

As I looked at the changes before me, I knew that this story of my early years in Harlem and the beginnings of Swing dance and the creation of Lindy Hop, and where jazz dance is today needed to be told, and I became determined to tell it.

I had been a part of that world, and, when it was over, I

was one of the dancers who made the transition into jazz dance. This book is about how I made a life in the world of Swing music and dance.

Coming to America

In 1915 fifteen year old Zalama Barker, my mother, landed at Ellis Island from Bridgetown, Barbados, certain that many opportunities awaited her.

After nearly two weeks on the ocean, most of the passengers had taken sick; steerage passengers had miserably hot and muggy accommodations, but to her the ship was a floating palace. She was on her way to New York—that magnificent city she had heard so much about was going to be her home. She was especially excited to see the place she had heard most about, the place where all of the colored people went—Harlem.

Zalama's heart was dancing. She was strong, young, and she was going to have a job where she would be on her own! No one was going to tell her where she could go or what she could do. Yes indeed, she was going to New York, and nothing could be better than that!

When they entered the harbor, she saw the Statue of Liberty, it seemed to be speaking to her, "Send me your tired, your poor, . . . yearning to be free." But, she wasn't tired, and she sure wasn't poor. Her sister Gwendolyn was waiting for her as was a job. That had been the plan: as the sisters came to America (there were three, Zalama being the second) they would save their money and send for the next sister. Her mother had planned this so that the family could relocate in America.

The plan seemed to be a good one, troubles didn't seem to exist. She had managed the entire trip without being sick, and she was far too excited to sleep, she was arriving in the land of opportunity.

After two days at Ellis Island, when she was finally allowed to leave, somehow her name had been changed to Alma. Zalama didn't argue about the name change, she was anxious to get out of Ellis Island and happy to be arriving in a new country.

Gwendolyn was waiting for her, and boy was she a sight for sore eyes! When she finally cleared customs, her sister whisked her away to that distant land called Brooklyn to see the other relatives who had preceded her, all asking questions about home. How was her mother, Carrie? How was her younger sister, Eunice, and when would she be coming?

Alma was also introduced to Mr. Nurse, the owner of the brownstone in which she would be living. Her sister and other immigrants already had rooms there. The system was that the tenants had rooms which they occupied one day a week, since their jobs were sleep–in positions with one day off. On that day they came home to settle their rent and the cost of their passage. It was like share cropping without farming, the immigrants were sent out to do housework in the homes of white people. Their job as a rule consisted of house–keeping, baby sitting, and a little cooking. Most families preferred to hire young girls so they could train them to cook, clean, and look after the children. All of these duties were explained to Alma; the fact that she was being exploited did not occur to her, she was still feeling the excitement of being in America. That night, after she was shown her room, she and Gwendolyn sat up talking about the family, and how they would bring Eunice over. Their hearts were full of hope. The future was bright, life was good.

The next day Alma was taken to the home of her new employers, the Goldfields. She was awed by the elegant wooden staircase and all of the beautiful shelves that lined the sitting room. She didn't realize that she would grow to despise all of that lovely wood; keeping it clean would be her most unpleasant duty.

This first day on the job she was taught how to clean a Jewish home. She was bewildered by the two sets of dishes and the way everything had to be scrubbed and scoured. After taking her through all of her household chores, Emma Goldfield, the lady of the house (who was not much older than Alma herself), showed her what she was expected to do for the baby. His name was Leo, and he was a very agreeable baby, rarely crying or fussing, and Alma grew to be quite fond of him. Mr. Goldfield arrived in the evening; he seemed to be a nice man but there was very little said between the two of them. He left all of the details of the new house girl to his wife.

Alma took her new job in stride. This was expected of her, and it was the only way she could repay the money spent on her passage and contribute to the passage for Eunice. Alma would be so pleased when Eunice could join her in America; they were the closest of the sisters. Gwendolyn, being the oldest, had responsibility for the

family in America. They had never been as close as she and
Eunice were, and with their present schedules, they could
see one another only once a week.

So, the land of opportunity wasn't all she had expected,
but it was a start. Her duties became routine, and she fit in
as best she could, doing everything possible to please her
employers.

Many times Alma found herself longing to be back
home. She missed her mother terribly, she missed the beach
that they used to play on, she missed the mangoes that she
and her sisters would pick off the trees, and she missed her
mother's cooking, oh how she longed for the taste of fungi
and fish, fresh from the sea.

Many nights she would lay in bed crying. It was then she
would remember her mother's words: "When you ain't got
a horse, ride a cow," and she'd fall off to sleep.

Nearly two years went by with very little change in
Alma's schedule. Six days a week she worked for the
Goldfields, and one day she had to herself to settle bills and
visit at the brownstone. When at last the money was paid
for Eunice to come, Alma was elated. She had missed her so
much during the two years since she left Barbados, she was
barely able to sleep the night before Eunice arrived.

The ship that carried Eunice to America arrived on
schedule, and both Alma and Gwendolyn were given the
day off to pick their sister up at Ellis Island. It was the first
time Alma had been to New York City since the day of her
own arrival. It was as crowded as she remembered, people
swarmed like angry hornets. It was a muggy day, and the
docks reeked of garlic as weary travelers left the ships
carrying their baskets and bundles. Travelers from the

islands were easy to spot—they carried straw bags as
luggage.

At last Alma spotted Eunice; and she and Gwendolyn
shouted to her at the top of their lungs. Just before they
both lost their voices, she saw them and neared the line at
the gate. It seemed to Alma that it took forever, for
Gwendolyn had to take care of the legal papers, but at long
last Eunice was released, and they were all together. They
hugged and cried, asking all of the questions about home,
exchanging news and dreams of the future.

Before Eunice had settled in her new home they received
the news that their mother had passed away while Eunice
was en route. The sisters were engulfed in emotion, the joy
of being together again and the sorrow of losing their
mother. They sat up reminiscing all night in a sort of
memorial for their mother. They were pleased that she had
accomplished what she had wanted most in life—her
daughters were in America, working toward better lives—
and they vowed that they would do everything to be a
credit to her memory; they were the Barkers of Barbados,
and whatever it took, they were going to make it!

NORMAN MILLER

Eunice had arrived in America just in time. The Lusitania had just been sunk and the papers were full of war news. Alma didn't think much about it. She was glad to have her sister there, but nothing was happening for her, she still wasn't going anywhere. Her chores were still the same, she hadn't gotten to New York on her own yet, and she hadn't seen Harlem.

Harlem was a dream for her, she had heard so much about it. It was where the colored people went, it was their own place. It had all the great dance halls, and it was where you could meet people from your own hometown. Mr. Nurse would bring the *Amsterdam News*, a newspaper that carried all the news about the people of Harlem, to the brownstone, and Alma would read it eagerly. Of course, Mr. Nurse tried to dissuade her from visiting Harlem saying, "It isn't a nice place for young single girls to go." That was all right for him to say, he thought she should stay in Brooklyn and do nothing but work to pay him rent and have no fun. She decided not to concern herself with what he wanted, she knew what she wanted, which was to go to Harlem and find a husband. Then she could get away from Mr. Nurse and his degrading brownstone!

It wasn't long before war was declared; it was the same week that she and Eunice made their first trip to Harlem. They didn't tell Gwendolyn who felt the same as Mr. Nurse.

It was a long ride, but Alma knew they would be fine as long as she remembered 135th Street and Lenox Avenue. The moment they emerged from the station, they were surrounded by people buzzing about America going to war. There were men on soap boxes telling the colored people they shouldn't enlist because of the way they were treated in America. "It's a white man's war, let them fight it." Alma was happy to be walking the streets of Harlem.

The people there were very easy to talk to. Alma felt a relaxed atmosphere that she had not experienced since coming to this country. Eunice, on the other hand, was a bit apprehensive, but she did enjoy the free feeling of touring the streets of Harlem. The sisters returned to Brooklyn at dark, but Alma knew she would be back.

The more they visited, the more they became familiar with the people and Harlem traditions. They were thrilled to learn of a Sons and Daughters of Barbados dance at Leroy's at 135th Street and 5th Avenue on the next Thursday, their one day off. They both loved to dance and were very interested in meeting eligible bachelors from their homeland.

The dance was crowded, but they didn't mind, the air was thick with their own familiar accent. As they stood against the wall waiting for an invitation to dance, Alma spied an especially handsome prospect. He was tall and dark with a smile that seemed to light up the whole room. She nearly blushed when he caught her looking at him. Embarrassed, she talked with Eunice, trying not to look at him again.

Before long the young man asked her to dance. Alma reluctantly replied that she didn't feel right leaving her sister

alone. The young man uttered something of an acceptance
and left. Alma was terribly disappointed. Still, she couldn't
leave her younger sister, who was already uncomfortable,
alone on the sidelines.

Alma and Eunice continued to stand against the wall.
Several melodies later, and feeling rather restless, Alma
suggested that they head for the early train and get home.
Eunice agreed, but as they approached the door, the handsome man touched Alma's arm. Another young man was
with him.

Alma was so taken by his grin that she did blush this time
but quickly regained her composure and introduced herself
and her sister. Norman Miller and his friend George asked
Alma and Eunice to dance. But Alma said that they had to
be going. Norman was difficult to discourage and Alma
stubbornly insisted they must leave. Although the young
men were making every effort to keep the girls from
leaving, Alma was playing hard to get.

As they left the dance and headed for the train, Alma
began to apologize for the young men's behavior, but
Eunice thought that Alma had been rude to the young men,
who were only trying to get them to do what they had
come there for—to dance!

Alma insisted that she was trying to preserve their dignity, but Eunice could not see how turning down a good
looking feller who was asking you to dance was preserving
dignity. Alma, secretly delighted, suggested maybe they
should give it another try the next week.

The following week they dressed carefully. Talk of the
young men filled their conversation until they arrived at the
dance, full of anticipation. The music had started, and Alma

almost immediately spotted Norman dancing with another
girl. Soon Norman approached them, smiled broadly, and
said he knew they couldn't stay away. He asked Alma if she
would like to dance, and this time there was no hesitation.
He led her to the center of the floor. She knew from
watching that he was a good dancer, but she hadn't realized
how good. Boy could he lead! Alma was delighted.

George caught up with Eunice, and both couples danced
nearly every dance. The night went by much too quickly,
but when it was over, the girls gave them their address at
the brownstone. George and Norman gave the girls direc-
tions to the room they shared. It was "real close" they said.
The girls thought it wasn't quite proper of them to have
invited them to their room so soon after meeting, but they
were flattered and talked of meeting again the next week.

All the way home Eunice and Alma chattered about the
fine prospects they had met. It was the first time Alma had
felt really happy since coming to America. The next week
her chores didn't seem so bad. She dreamt of the next
Thursday and of Norman and the next dance with him.

The girls went the next week and the next and the next.
Eunice met a number of young men and enjoyed dancing
with all of them. Alma, on the other hand, was more than
content to dance only with Norman. They seemed insepa-
rable; Alma and Norman were falling in love.

Sometime later Eunice announced to Alma that she
wouldn't be going to Harlem that night because she had too
much to do at the brownstone. When Alma pressed her
sister for a better explanation, Eunice admitted that she was
just tired of watching the two lovebirds every week, and she
was jealous that she didn't have a special man of her own.

Alma argued she sure wasn't going to find a husband sitting
at home, but Eunice could not be swayed. So, Alma went
to Leroy's alone. Norman was there, and they danced and
talked all night long. He was surprised to see her there
alone, but didn't mind in the least; he saw this as an opportunity and suggested she take the late train home. They
could stop at his place on the way to the station. Alma
wanted to go to his room, she wasn't ready to go home yet.
She was nervous but heard herself saying that it was a nice
idea, and they started up the block to Norman's place.

When they got to the room, Alma saw that it wasn't
much. It was furnished with only two beds and a small
dresser. The room's modesty surprised her, after all Norman
was a sharply dressed man. Norman sat on his bed and
patted the vacant space next to him, asking her to have a
seat and insisting that he wouldn't bite.

It was just seconds before their mouths were locked and
not much longer before their feet moved from the floor to
the bed. Then he told her he loved her. Alma thought her
heart would burst with joy, and she told him that she loved
him too.

Norman kissed her softly on her forehead, then her
eyelids, her cheeks, Alma could only lie there with her eyes
closed and wonder what wonderful thing would happen
next. She thought of Carrie, her mother, and wondered
what would she think? A single girl in a man's room, not
wanting it to end. Certainly if they were in love that made
it okay.

Her racing thoughts were interrupted by Norman's
voice. It sounded small, almost reverent, he was asking her
if she had ever been with a man before. She replied that of

NORMAN MILLER

course she had not, she had never felt this way before. Alma surrendered her body to him, she could not imagine leaving now. Moments later they lay there, neither knowing what to say. Alma was blissfully happy to be there in his arms, yet she felt ashamed, she could not look at Norman. Then, stroking her forehead, he asked if she was all right. She looked up into his eyes and knew that she was.

As they walked toward the station they talked very little. When they arrived Norman kissed her gently on the cheek and promised to see her the next Thursday.

The ride home seemed especially long, and the next morning Eunice asked why she had been so late the night before. She said she missed her train and left it at that. She couldn't possibly tell her sister what she had done.

The weekly visits to Harlem and the dances continued, but Alma did not return to Norman's room. She couldn't without making Eunice suspicious. Actually it was a good excuse for Alma. Although Norman had mentioned marriage he had not proposed, and she certainly did not want to put herself in that situation with him again when he might not ever become her husband.

One morning as Alma started her day at the Goldfields' she began feeling very ill. She stood polishing the wood on the stairs, and the smell of the polish nearly made her wretch. She sat down for a moment to get a breath, and Mrs. Goldfield came around the corner. Seeing Alma she asked if she was okay. Alma explained that she hadn't slept well the night before, and she was sure she would be fine in a minute.

Alma's chores became increasingly difficult. She felt tired all of the time. Mrs. Goldfield became concerned. She was a kind woman, and she didn't want to lose Alma as a house girl, she was a good worker. Finally Mrs. Goldfield suggested she go to the clinic.

It was a hot August day, the waiting room was full of coughing people and crying babies. There was no chair available and she felt sure she would faint from the heat. At last they called her name and she went into the examination room. The doctor began asking a string of questions and finally asked if she was having intercourse. When she answered that she had one time, he called a nurse to draw blood. When Alma asked why, the nurse said that the doctor thought she might be having a baby. Alma's head was swimming. Pregnant? No, that could not happen to her. Surely she just had the flu or a cold. Maybe she had eaten some bad meat.

Alma was asked to come back the next day for the test results but said she could not come back until her day off. The next Thursday she got the results. She was pregnant.

That evening she had very little to say as she and Eunice prepared to leave for Harlem. Norman met them at the station as he had been doing, and they made small talk as they headed for Leroy's.

The last dance of the night was a slow dance, and Norman was holding her closely. She could hardly stand it, how was she going to tell him? Then, when he mentioned slipping off to his room, she blurted out that that was how she had gotten into this mess, that she was pregnant! She stood rigid as stone in his arms.

His reply was not what she had expected; he said that it was wonderful news! He was rambling in his excitement, telling her that they could get married and she would move to Harlem. They would raise the baby there. He couldn't wait for them to be a family! Everything seemed to be working out better than she had hoped.

Norman made her promise that she would wait a week before telling anyone. He said the next week they would make plans; he would propose properly, and then they'd tell everybody!

The next Thursday Norman was not waiting for them at the station. Occasionally he worked late and would just meet them at the dance, but when they got to the dance he was no where to be seen. Eight o'clock came, no Norman. Nine o'clock. Ten o'clock. The dance was over and he had not come! At first Alma was angry, then she began to worry. What if he was sick? She begged Eunice to stop at his room before going to the subway. No one was there.

As they headed for the station, Alma thought her legs would give out. They felt like rubber, she felt sick to her stomach. Moments later she was crying.

Eunice turned to comfort her, insisting that there was a simple explanation. She would see him next week. Then Alma told her sister that she was pregnant and that he must not want her or their baby!

Eunice was shocked and happy and sad all at once. A baby was a great thing, but having no husband was a problem. And what was she going to tell Gwendolyn?

Telling Gwendolyn was no easy task, but together they mustered the courage and went to her. They were surprised by her reaction. She didn't get angry at Alma and said they had to stick together, because they were all each other had.

Alma went to work the next day heart sick. Nothing made sense anymore, what would she do when the baby came? Who would take care of them? Surely her job at the Goldfield's would come to an end. Things could not be worse for her, but every day she remembered to thank God, at least she had her sisters.

Months later she lay in her room at the brownstone on her day off when Eunice came in with a letter from Norman!

He had been drafted. He was there waiting at the station for them when they took him. He and many other men had been conscripted, herded like cattle and shipped off directly to boot camp. He hadn't even been given the chance to contact her until then. He still wanted to marry her! Until then the war had meant very little to Alma.

Plans were made for them to see one another on his first furlough. Before he could get there, Alma found herself in labor. She was taken to St. Michael's hospital where Dorothy Barker was born on March 7, 1918.

When Norman got back they were married immediately. The sisters and the happy couple had a small family celebration, and Alma and Dorothy Barker became Alma and Dorothy Miller. Too quickly Norman had to return to service.

November 11, 1918, Armistice Day was a happy day for everyone, and no one was happier than Alma. The soldiers would be returning soon, and she would be moving to Harlem with her husband and their baby. When Norman returned she got her wish, she could now call Harlem her home.

The apartment they took was small, but it was a happy home. Alma was blissful, she was able to stay home and raise her baby while Norman worked in the shipyards of Brooklyn. By March Alma announced they were going to have another baby. Norman didn't mind, he loved being a papa. Even though he spent most of his time working, the little time he spent with his family was the best time of his life. He had always wanted a big family of his own. Money could never be so tight that he wouldn't want more children.

By October Norman contracted pneumonia from the damp conditions at the shipyards. Before long he was hospitalized, developed double pneumonia, and Alma was summoned to come immediately.

Eunice made the long subway trip to the veteran's hospital with Alma who was eight months pregnant. When they arrived Norman was very weak. He died within the hour leaving his young family with no insurance and no means of support.

December 2, 1919, Norma Miller was born, one month after her father's death. Alma's sisters pitched in whenever they could so she could survive until she could get a job, but it was difficult to get work with two small children; the day nurseries would not take an infant. The church helped in a small way too. Someone suggested that she put her children in an orphanage until she could get back on her feet. Having no choice, Alma packed her children's few belongings and took them to the orphanage. As the attendant explained the process to her, a little girl pulled on her skirt and asked if Alma was her mama. Suddenly Alma could see her little Dot wandering around the orphanage, wondering who her mama was. She made a decision then and there. "I've changed my mind. I'll suck salt before I ever leave my children in any orphanage, I'll never separate us ever!" and with that she left. She kept that vow until her dying day.

THE EARLY YEARS

I made my debut in the world with a lot of strikes against me. With no father and Mama struggling to survive, it's a wonder we made it at all. My aunts would look down at me lying in my crib and say, "Oh that poor child, she's got no father and she looks just like a bunny rabbit." (The nick name, Bunny stuck permanently.) What we did have going for us was that Mama was a fighter. She was willing to do whatever it took to get us by, and she did.

It was 1920, the birth of the Jazz Age. People were dancing the Charleston, women wore stockings rolled to their knees, bootleg whiskey was everywhere, and Harlem saw the arrival of black people from the South in droves. They were looking for a place to feel this new freedom. Although West Indians still flocked to Brooklyn, Mama wanted Harlem to be her home; it was where she belonged.

The first apartment I can remember was at 139th Street and Lenox Avenue. The music we heard all around us was this new jazz. Part of Mama's survival technique was to give house rent parties. She would have cards printed up to announce them. They would be held on Saturday nights, the admission price was twenty–five cents, and the money she raised would be used to pay the rent. Mama would sell pigs feet, peas and rice, and jump steady (another name for bootleg whiskey). Guests would flock to our apartment, and dance the famous Charleston, which I learned by watching them. Before long I became the entertainment. I would fall asleep on the pile of coats in the bedroom, and Mama would wake me to perform. I loved the attention, and when Mama threw in the extra incentive of ice cream, I could dance all night.

Throughout the 1920s the migration to Harlem continued. People came from the North, the South, the Caribbean. There were artists, writers, painters, and hustlers. Mama seemed to befriend them all. This eclectic group offered an endless variety of views and opinions. Mama had always been a rebel, and she was certainly open to anything that might lead her to a better way of life.

When one of my aunts was available to sit for us, Mama would go to the corners in the Bronx at which people picked up day workers to clean their homes. Survival was always an issue for the black family, and Mama did everything she could to see that we survived.

One evening Mama came home from her days work quite late, and told Gwen she had been to see a man named Marcus Garvey who was speaking at the hall. He'd said he was going to change things, that he had started a shipping line for Negroes, and we could invest in it, make a lot of money, and then move to Africa where we would be treated like first–class citizens. It was called the Black Star Line, and we could buy in for only five dollars a share—we would own part of the company.[1] She told Gwen that she had to get a uniform, too, because she planned to march for Garvey! She insisted that they all had to go and see him next time he spoke.

Gwen was speechless. She could not believe that Mama

[1] *The African American Encyclopedia*, Vol. 3, s.v. Marcus Garvey, 645.

could honestly consider paying this man money when she could barely keep a roof over our heads.

Mama argued that it was for a better life. She told Gwen that we were never going to be more than slaves to white folks, that we needed to get out of this country and make a better life for ourselves. She asked Gwen if she didn't have faith in her own kind. Gwen answered that she would talk to Mama when she was making more sense, gathered her things, and left.

Mama managed to come up with the three dollars to purchase her uniform. It was all white with a ribbon across the chest, and she did march for Marcus Garvey.

Gwendolyn and Eunice did manage to talk Mama out of being a Garvyite—Mama was always more of an enlistee than an activist. They argued that they had already traveled all this way from the West Indies; what good could it possibly do to pack up and move to Africa? After all, they were already in the land of freedom. The decision was made, and the Barker sisters decided to stay in America and fight the fight for freedom in New York.

By 1922 it seemed that Marcus Garvey was the con man that Eunice and Gwendolyn believed him to be. He was charged with fraud by the federal government.[2] Mama, however, who felt the whole arrest was a plot by the government, continued to believe in him. She had simply chosen to stay in America.

The Harlem Renaissance continued in full force. As the migration to Harlem increased, so did the goings on in the streets. Mama wanted Dot and me to have a structured life, she didn't want us growing up in the streets of Harlem. So,

[2] *The African American Encyclopedia*, Vol. 3, s.v. Amy Jacques Garvey, 643.

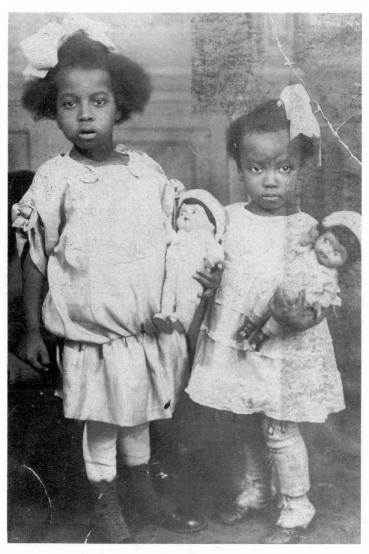

Norma Miller (right), *at age 3 and her sister, Dorothy Miller* (left),
at age 5, in 1923.

from the first summer I can remember, she managed to get us into summer camp. We would go to Camp Schermerhorn at Milford, Connecticut. It was a program set up by St. Phillip's Church for poor children and their mothers to have two weeks together at camp each summer.

Mama would work magic, after the two weeks at Camp Schermerhorn we would be sent directly to Camp Minisink. We would spend nearly the entire summer at camp. Rather than cavorting through the streets of Harlem during those sweltering months, we were chaperoned. We would make crafts and swim, and I always did a lot of dancing. Boy how I loved to entertain. Some of the girls and I would put together acts and perform for the whole camp. Mama, God bless her, always encouraged me.

One summer when we returned from camp, we moved to 142nd Street off of Lenox Avenue, right across the street from the Cotton Club. It was my last summer of freedom, I was to start school in the Fall. It was a mystical summer, I was so excited about the school year that lay ahead of me, yet I didn't want the summer to end. The windows of the Cotton Club were open every night, and we could hear the beautiful music played by the Duke Ellington Band. We could look out and see the show from a distance. I was overwhelmed by the music and the desire to dance, some-how I knew that I was going to be in show business.

Fall soon swallowed up the long summer nights, and I was enrolled at P.S. 139. It was right across the street from where we lived, and it was the happiest day of my young life. Dot had already started school, and it had been very lonely for me without her. At last I was going to be able to play with other children. I arrived my first day in a crisp new dress, a new pair of shiny black patent–leather shoes, and a big bow in my hair. I strutted into the classroom like a peacock!

I continued to show an interest in dance, so Mama signed me up for Saturday dance classes. There was nothing I would rather do than dance, and when my class was over I would stay and watch the next classes. I would stay all day long just watching and practicing.

In my fourth year of school I was transferred to P.S. 90 at 147th Street between 7th and 8th Avenue, and I could go by myself. I know Mama was relieved to have Dot and me getting ourselves to school so that she could go to work without worrying about us. It was at P.S. 90 that my interest in music and dance truly blossomed. The movie musicals were the highlight of our conversations every Monday. I tried to memorize all the dance numbers that I had seen in the movies, and I knew all the songs. The Charleston was the big dance, and we would try all the new steps in the school gym: the Black Bottom, the Shimmy, Picking Cherries, and a new dance that they were doing in the Cotton Club show called the Shim Sham. Betty, a friend of mine, and I would get together and practice. Her mother was in the chorus line at the Cotton Club, and Betty had learned the Shim Sham from her; I learned it from Betty. That day I danced those steps all the way home, and I never forgot them.

THE SAVOY

With 1929 came the Great Depression, and my family's struggle for survival got tougher. Mama usually held us together with the courage of an army general, but no one can be strong all of the time. One unbearably cold winter's day, when the sky was black with clouds and the wind was screaming through our poorly insulated walls, Dot and I sat huddled in a blanket in the bedroom, and we heard Aunt Eunice rush through the door. I heard Mama tell her to shut the door before we froze to death, say it was a hell of a day to be out visiting, and ask if her being there meant she got the money to help us out with the rent. Aunt Eunice sounded upset when she told Mama she was sorry, that she had asked Gwen but she didn't have much, and she couldn't come up with the rest. Mama's voice sounded strange. She was very quiet, and she told Eunice she understood, but she guessed we'd be moving again. She mumbled something about how she sure didn't know who was gonna take the three of us for what she could pay them, but she would work it out. She told Eunice she was tired and needed to get some rest. Eunice whispered another apology, and I heard the door open and then close behind her.

I could hear Mama muttering to herself. I barely recognized her voice. I peaked around the corner. The room was growing dark, and Mama hadn't turned on any lights. I saw her putting something on the Victrola, and then I heard   the voice of Bessie Smith singing about being poor and lonesome; singing about how doing right doesn't get you treated right. As the light left the room, I listened to Bessie wailing on the Victrola and knew that Mama was crying too.

Languishing in her own depression was not Mama's style. When morning came, the sun was shining, the wind had died down, and the only screaming we heard was Mama's voice announcing we were moving.

She told us we were outta the damned place, she had never liked it, and it was time to move on. She said the walls weren't much thicker than a cardboard box, and she must've been a damned fool to pay them to live in such a hole! She told us what was to be packed and what would be left behind, and she said she would be back that afternoon to collect us. By evening we were in our new apartment. It was a third floor apartment on 140th Street and the fire escape window faced the back of the Savoy ballroom.

The Savoy had opened three years earlier in flush times. Prohibition was still the law in 1926, but enforcement was easing now that the city cops had decided to leave it to the feds. Nightclubs were coming back again; the Cotton Club, Small's Paradise, and Connie's Inn were the most popular new clubs. Harlem was becoming the entertainment capitol of the world. At night, Society came to Harlem, they called it slumming. These clubs regularly would be filled with an exclusively white clientele who enjoyed the entirely black entertainment. White people owned Harlem; it was said that Harlem was for the Negroes in the A.M. but for the whites in the P.M.

The real upsurge in Harlem night life was triggered by the opening, on March 12, 1926, of Harlem's most elegant ballroom—the Savoy. The Savoy was built for black patrons; there was no separate entrance for whites, there were no balconies where the white customers would watch the blacks perform. The opening of the Savoy marked a change in the social pattern. For the first time in history, the status quo in America was challenged. At last there was a beautiful ballroom with no segregation. Black people and white people danced on the same dance floor, they sat and ate across from one another in the booths; everyone's money was the same at the Savoy.

Once the Savoy opened, others did as well. After-hour joints were kinds of uptown speakeasies, and Harlem was crawling with them. It was the place to go to get anything you wanted, especially if it was illegal. The Cotton Club was near the Savoy at 142nd Street and Lenox Avenue. When people left the Cotton Club, a stop at the Savoy was a must. You could club crawl until the wee hours of the morning in Harlem.

The Savoy occupied the entire city block from 140th to 141st Streets, and overnight it became Harlem's landmark. From the beginning the Savoy was the largest and most elegant ballroom in Harlem. It's fame soon spread, across the country and throughout the world.

Whether you drove or took a bus up Lenox Avenue you couldn't miss the huge Savoy marquee advertising the bands that would vie for the favor of the evening's audience. Entering the Savoy one was met by the doorman, "Big

George" Calleaux, an ex–prize fighter from New Orleans.
Big George wore diamonds up and down his tuxedo shirt
and a big diamond ring on his pinky finger. Single women
knew they would be able to leave the Savoy safely, as he
would see that they got into a taxi without being bothered.
Nobody messed with Big George.

Ticket's were sold at the booth beneath the marquee. It
cost thirty cents before six P.M., sixty cents between six and
eight P.M., and eighty–five cents after eight.[1] On entering
you went down a flight of stairs to check your coat with
Mr. Charles Parkinson, who ran the check stand for
twenty–five years, then up two flights of marble stairs,
between walls lined with mirrors to the ballroom.

At the top of the stairs the Savoy's unobtrusive security
force discreetly kept track of the patrons. Jack La Rue, a
massive man with lethal hands, a huge head, and brawny
shoulders, directed the four men who covered the ballroom
each night. He kept his staff moving inconspicuously
throughout the evening and usually posted someone near
the top of the stairs to keep out prostitutes, drunks, and any
man not wearing a jacket and tie.

The ballroom itself was decorated in gold and blue and
illuminated with colored spotlights. The walls were lined
with booths for eating and drinking. The dance area was
fifty feet by two hundred feet, the length of a city block.
The dance floor itself was made of many layers of hard-
wood, such as mahogany and maple. By mid–evening,
when the band was swinging and the place was jumping
with dancers, you could feel the floor beneath you undulating

[1] Helen Clarke, Savoy hostess, personal interview, 1984.

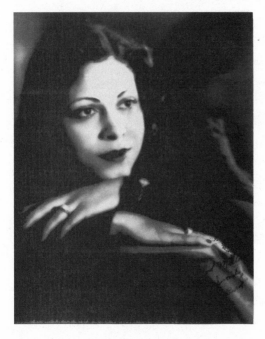

Cissy Bowe, a hostess at the Savoy.

"In those days if you were dark you couldn't get into a chorus line. Hostesses at the Savoy had to be good dancers, well dressed, and follow the rules. Anyone who broke the rules about not socializing with the customers would be fined."

with their movement. It was replaced every three years, worn out from the constant pounding.

To the right of the entrance was another ticket booth, nearby a set of chairs occupied by some of the most exquisite women around. These were the Savoy Hostesses, well known as Harlem's most beautiful women. You could purchase a dance with them at this ticket booth for a quarter; they would even teach you to dance if need be. But

they were forbidden to see patrons outside of the Savoy,
doing so would cost them their jobs.

Music at the Savoy never stopped. There were two,
sometimes three bandstands, and one of them was jumping
anytime the ballroom was open. The bandstand on the 141st
Street side would be occupied by the house band, while the
other would be given to one or another of the traveling
bands that happened to be in town. Whenever one band
was about to end its set, the other would jump in on the
final chorus and then take off on its own.

The Savoy opened with two bands: Fess Williams and his
Royal Flush Orchestra and Duncan Mayer's Savoy Bearcats.
Williams, a flashy band leader known for his top hat and his
shimmering diamond studded tuxedo, would achieve
national fame as the first house band of the Savoy. In the

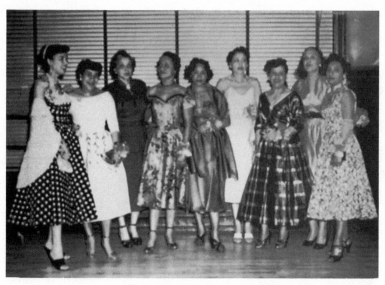

Helen Clarke (second from left), a hostess at the Savoy, photographed in the 1950s.

"Cab was the swingin'est there ever was. He was my inspiration in show business. I'll never forget when I saw him make his entrance on stage at the Apollo Theater: he came down a long staircase wearing a big cape with rhinestones and a top hat, and when he opened the cape he was wearing a white coat with tails. He was just fabulous."

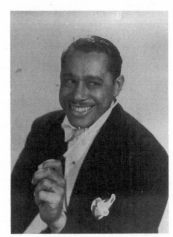

Cab Calloway.

years to follow, over two hundred and fifty of the best jazz bands in the world would appear at the Savoy.

Jazz needed a place to develop where innovation was not only accepted but was encouraged; indeed, where those who were timid were left behind. That place was the Savoy. It was where white and black musicians mixed. With the exception of Cab Calloway and later Duke Ellington, it wasn't until late in the Swing Era, in the late 1930s, that black bands could play for the white clientele in hotels and other ballrooms. But since audiences wanted to hear Cab Calloway, not the band behind him, the soloists were not spotlighted. Most of the innovative work came from black bands like those led by Jimmie Lunceford and Lucky Millinder who were restricted to playing in the poorer paying clubs in black areas. But everyone was comfortable at the Savoy.

"LUCKY WAS SeCONd ONly to CAB AS A Big BANd leAdeR. He ReAlly
pumped it up, As the kids say today. He dANced while he led
the bANd, ANd his coAt tAils SwuNg iN RhythM with the music.
MilliNdeR iNtRoduced SisteR RosettA ThARpe to the SAvoy."

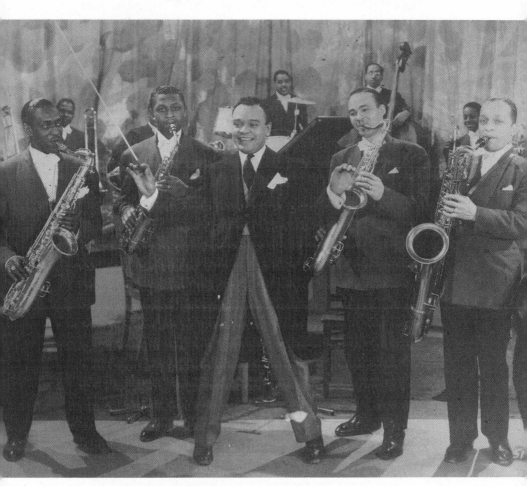

Lucky Millinder and his band.

Benny Goodman, for instance, played the Savoy only once—during his famous battle of the bands with Chick Webb in 1938. However, he visited often when he was in New York and was invited to sit in with the band on numerous occasions, as were the Dorseys and numerous sidemen in white bands.

Many a famous singer got started at the Savoy as well. In 1934, for instance, Chick Webb plucked the young Ella Fitzgerald out of an Apollo engagement and groomed her for his band. Lena Horne earned much of her early acclaim at the Savoy, as did Billie Holiday, Dinah Washington, and Sarah Vaughan. Frank Sinatra, the Andrews Sisters, Jo Stafford, Jimmy Rushing, and others sang there.

The Savoy played an enormous and largely unrecognized role in the history of jazz. The Savoy should always be remembered along with the men and women who created the music that all America danced to. The musicians who produced Swing; Goodman, Ellington, Henderson, Webb, Moten, Waller, Miller, Basie, Lunceford, James, and hundreds of other composers, arrangers, and instrumentalists deserve the admiration and respect of all who love good music.

The effects of the Depression continued to ravage our community and our family. Mama, being a black woman, was unable to get a steady job. In fact, most black workers had lost their regular jobs when the Depression hit. Employers tended to keep their white employees in hard times, and the effects were devastating. Blacks were last to be hired, first to be fired. Mama would go to the corners to be hired for daily domestic work, but competition for any income was stiff, and often she would take a days work for ten cents an hour.

Gwendolyn and Eunice were having their own money troubles and could rarely help us out. There was no public welfare system at the time, and Mama, being a widowed mother of two, had to turn to the church for support. We were long–time members of the St. Phillip's Church congregation and they always did what they could to help. Unfortunately, there were hundreds of other families in need as well. The relief lines were long, and the available assistance was limited, but Mama swallowed her pride and did everything she could to keep a roof over our heads and food in our bellies. During this time she learned that the all–black Abyssinian Baptist Church was offering assistance to any family that needed it. Although we were Episcopalian, we were welcome there. This was how Mama discovered the young assistant pastor of the church, Adam Clayton Powell, Jr. Being a politically minded woman, she was immediately drawn to him. She actually attended a Baptist service to hear him speak. He was a flamboyant man and a powerful orator, speaking out for the black community, which was also Mama's passion.

It was at this church that she learned that five black doctors lost their jobs at Harlem Hospital because five white doctors needed positions. The doctors asked Powell to help them regain their positions. As they explained their situation to Powell, he became furious. He recognized that the same thing was happening at all employment levels in Harlem. Black citizens were losing their jobs so that the whites wouldn't be unemployed. He knew that his church was struggling to feed so many hungry black families, not simply because of the Depression, but also because of the unfairness and prejudice of the employers. Powell immediately

mobilized the community and formed the Committee on
Harlem Hospital. He met with every official who would see
him and kept up the picketing. Night after night Mama,
who spent as much time picketing as she could spare, would
come home dispirited. They were not being taken seriously.
When it became clear that this approach was not working,
Powell and the Committee called for a mass protest. He
realized that the only power blacks had in the community
was their numbers, and if he organized enough of them in
one demonstration he could get the attention needed to
start making changes.

In Spring 1931, churches announced the planned protest,
and signs were posted throughout the community. Still,
there were no guarantees that any supporters would attend,
and it was feared that the presence of hundreds of riot
police, positioned directly in front of City Hall, might scare
off potential demonstrators. But a flood of supporters began
to arrive. By the time the crowd had fully assembled there
were about six thousand people marching together.[2] The
significance of this demonstration opened the doors to a
meeting of the Board of Estimate that was in session. Powell
was able to tell them of the situation in the hospital and, as a
result, Harlem Hospital policy was completely rewritten.
Adam Clayton Powell, Jr., was giving hope back to our
community and back to our family. Mama was very proud
to have taken part in the movement and to have a new
figure in Harlem worthy of her support.

Soon the sun came and melted away the remains of

[2] Haskins, James S., *Adam Clayton Powell: Portrait of a Marching Black*. (Trenton, N.J.: Africa World Press, 1993), 30.

winter. At last Dot and I were free to play outside. The neighborhood was full of children many of whom, like myself, loved to dance. Although Dot refused to join in because she thought we looked ridiculous, the rest of us would hang around outside the Savoy and dance to the music that spilled out of the ballroom. We were always being chased off by the doormen. But minutes later we'd be back on the sidewalk. Eventually they would tire of yelling at us and let us be. Appreciative passersby would actually throw pennies to us as we danced. We would stop and scramble to pick them up, arguing over whom they were actually throwing the money at. These were the Depression years and money was tight in our neighborhood, anything that could buy a movie ticket or a piece of candy was precious property.

As the weather turned hot and we were released from school for the summer Dot and I would spend evenings on the fire escape, listening to the music that filtered through the open windows of the ballroom. I would say, "One of these days I'm gonna go in there and dance the night away." We often were rocked to sleep by a swinging lullaby, and I'd dream about walking into that ballroom and being swept off my feet by a handsome man.

I remember Easter Sunday, 1932; the minute church let out I ran to the ballroom. Although there was an Easter Parade in Harlem, just like the one on Fifth Avenue, for me the real parade was going on at the Savoy Ballroom. The music had started and we kids gathered on the sidewalk as usual and began to dance. I heard someone calling out, "Hey kid!"

I turned, pointed to myself, and answered, "Who me?"

"Yeah, you kid, c'mere." He gestured with his head for me to come over. I could only stare, I was flabbergasted.

Finally I coaxed my legs into moving. I went over as if in a trance. I knew who he was immediately, everyone knew him. It was the greatest dancer at the Savoy, Twist Mouth George. As I walked over I could see where his name came from; the bizarre smile was on the side of his face. He was dressed in white from head to toe. Suit, hat, tie, and shoes. His hat was cocked to the side of his face where the twist was, and he had the longest pair of legs I had ever seen. He was clean from head to toe, man he was sharp.

He took my hand and said, "Listen kid, you look like a good dancer, how would you like to dance with me?"

I stared at him and could hardly speak. "You mean me? Me dance with you? When? Where?" I almost yelled the words, "Yes! Yes!" I said it a couple of times to be sure he heard me. There could be no doubts, to dance with Twist Mouth George. Wow!

He gestured toward the ballroom. "This afternoon for the Easter matinée, I think you would be a surprise to them. Would you like to do it?" I nodded yes. He patted my hand as if to reassure me, and said, "Wait here, I'll be right back." He walked over to the doorman Big George and gestured toward me. I saw Big George look back. I wondered what he thought, I knew he considered me a pest. Whatever went down, when Twist Mouth walked back he was still smiling.

He said, "It's all right for you to go in, but I got to be responsible for you, so you got to get out right after the contest. Okay?"

"Okay!" I promised. I almost jumped for joy. I was going

to go into the Savoy. Yipes! He told me he would come
back to fetch me when it was time, and he went back inside
the ballroom.

I waited on the same spot, not daring to leave for fear of
missing him when he came to get me. At last I saw him
come back out of the doors, he came to me and took my
hand. I had to run to keep up with him, we took the steps
two at a time. I was breathless when I walked into the
ballroom. He was moving so fast, and I was trying to take it
all in. It was the most beautiful place I had ever seen. The
soft lights, the music coming over the whole place, and
everywhere I looked there were people dancing close
together, holding hands, or walking together. I had stepped
into a romantic paradise.

Twist Mouth guided me to one of the booths, way back
in the corner and said, "Now you sit here and wait. I'll
come and get you when it's time for you to dance. Would
you like a Coca-Cola? I'll have the waiter bring you a
Coke," he said as he walked away. I just sat there trying to
take in every detail. I wanted to be sure this moment would
last me a long time.

Soon people were asked to clear the floor, and they
settled down around the edges, leaving the center open for
the parade and show. After the floor was cleared, a tall,
distinguished West Indian with cropped, greying hair and a
professional air came through the center and announced the
parade. He was Mr. Charles Buchanan, manager of the
Savoy. The parade was snappy and full of brilliant colors.
The winners were picked, and the time came for the
dancers to begin. This was not a dancing contest, but a
dancing show held for the matinée, and our appearance was

the surprise of the show. Twist Mouth brought me to the floor. People were staring and wondering what a mere child was doing on the dance floor. Twist Mouth took my hand when they announced, "Twist Mouth and his new partner!"

He looked at me, patted my hand and said, "Don't worry, just follow me and you'll be okay."

As we made our first swing–out, it seemed that Twist Mouth just lifted me in the air. My feet felt like they never touched the floor. People roared and at the end we did a step called a flying jig walk. The house came down. At the finish, Twist Mouth hoisted me onto his shoulders and paraded me around the floor. People were smiling and patting Twist Mouth on the back. I could hear them saying, "Twist Mouth is always coming up with something different." "That was too much Twist Mouth."

There is nothing more expressive than Harlem when they love you, and they loved George "Twist Mouth" Ganaway. He carried me all the way to the door, put me down, and thanked me. Then he bussed me on the cheek and led me out of the ballroom. I was as happy as a kid could be. I danced all the way home.

"Whee, wait 'til I tell them" I thought. But after thinking it over I decided not to tell Mama and Dot, they wouldn't believe me anyway. They thought I was a borderline nut, so I decided it best to keep it as my own secret. I was thrilled. I had just danced with Twist Mouth George. He thought I was a good dancer. That night, I went to bed with sugar plums in my head. I had danced in the world's most famous ballroom—the Savoy! And I had danced with the most famous of dancers—Twist Mouth George!

Coming of Age

In the fall of 1932, I started junior high school at P.S. 136,
a new school at 135th Street. We had to wear a uniform,
a white middy blouse and a tie; the color of your tie indi-
cated the grade you were in.

Mama was working in the laundry of the Harlem Hospital (a possible result of the Adam Clayton Powell efforts),
and she would do our middy blouses at work. Dot and I
went to school everyday in a newly starched uniform.
Nothing looked better than to see groups of girls in the halls
with sparkling uniforms, white and crispy. We were very
proud of the way we looked when we went to school.

I stayed at P.S. 136 for a year and a half before I learned of
P.S. 89, where they had a better music program. With my
love of music and dance, Mama allowed me to transfer
there. At P.S. 89 I took music appreciation. Mrs. Jones was
our teacher and she truly loved music and children. She
introduced us to all the classics: Mozart, Bach, Beethoven.
. . . They surely enriched our lives, but, being kids, we
were more interested in Swing. Mrs. Jones didn't object;
she formed a student choir and encouraged us to be creative. We took the assigned songs and gave them a beat. As
part of a contest with the other (white) junior high schools
we sang "Liberty Bell," which we had altered just a bit. We
made it swing!

Liberty Bell, a voice resounding
Ringing your message clear and strong!
Ringing of liberty, peace, and freedom
And the right ever conquer wrong!
Liberty Bell, Liberty Bell
Ring the song you sing so well
Liberty Bell, Liberty Bell
Ring, Ring
Liberty Bell
Ringing of freedom, Let your voices swell
Swing, Ring forever, Liberty Bell
Ring out!

We were just doing what came naturally, and our school took second place.

The school principal was Mrs. Johnson, and she took special notice of me. I suppose she recognized my talent and wanted to motivate me in the right direction. I was invited to accompany her to a number of after–school events; dance and music performances. I already knew that dancing was going to be an important part of my life. I had passed the local dancing school level, but at the time ballet and pro-gressive–dance classes weren't available to poor black children. So, a dance career seemed only a dream.

Swing music had become the music of our generation. There was a local ballroom called the Renaissance, at 138th Street and 7th Avenue which had matinées for young people. One Sunday after church I was hanging out with a couple of the guys I knew from 140th Street. They were telling me about these dances, and my friend Raddie sug-gested we go check out the "Renny." It was the first I'd

heard of this, and it sounded great to me. I was even dressed
for the occasion. I was wearing a pink organdy dress and
black patent–leather Cuban heels. Unfortunately, I had one
problem; I didn't have the twenty–five cents for admission.
The boys dug deep into their pockets and chipped in to pay
my way. When we got to the Renny I was so excited I
could hardly wait in line. It was the first time I had ever
gone into a ballroom as a patron. To think, I was going to
be able to dance all I wanted and see the band right up
close! The band was Vernon Andrade's, the band for us
kids.

It was the first time I would dance the Lindy, the dance I
had been watching at the Savoy from our fire escape. It was
exciting, energetic, and definitely my kind of dance. While
I was dancing, my sister Dot called my name. She was not
pleased to see me there. I told her that Raddie and the
fellers had brought me there, but she didn't want to hear it.
The feller dancing with her pleaded my case, saying I
seemed to be having a good time. She said that I was only
twelve years old and had no business being there. Finally we
agreed that I'd go straight home after the dance, and then
we would talk. I would have promised anything to keep on
dancing.

Music was never difficult for me to hear, and I began to
understand its rhythms. Suddenly, the dancing on the street,
the dances I had learned at school, all came together. I
danced every dance at the Renny that day.

The matinée lasted until six o'clock, and, as I promised, I
headed straight home, I wanted to be sure to get there
before Dot did. When she got home she called,

"Bunny . . ."

"I'm here. See, I promised I'd come straight home, and I did."

"I don't want to see you up there again, and if I do catch you I'm going to tell Mama."

"Oh, okay, I promise."

I lied. I had my fingers crossed behind me, it was one promise I had no intention of keeping.

I loved the music, and I loved the dancing, the Lindy Hop was one swinging dance. This was the way to a dancing career. I began to live for Sundays at the Renny. All week long I would think up schemes to get twenty–five cents and get out of the house on Sunday afternoon. Eventually, Dot got used to the idea and quit nagging me about not going. Sonny Ashby was my partner, and our best friend, Billy Leech, would go with us every week. There were other talented young dancers at the Renny too. There was Frankie Manning who was innovative and smooth. There was also William Downes and his sister Joyce. They became so good at the Lindy Hop that, although they were only twelve and thirteen years old, they would dance at other ballrooms too. Many of the dancers from the Renny eventually became my colleagues in the dance world.

We spent years at the Renny, practicing the craft that had become my passion. Eventually we learned of contests all over Harlem. The contests were so popular that they began springing up everywhere, overflowing into the theaters and nightclubs. The theaters had realized that the contests were a shot in the arm for their business. One contest in particular, the Savoy Lindy Hop Contest really caught our attention.

One of these contests was being held at the Apollo

theater. Ralph Cooper, the emcee, had started the contest to bring in business on Thursdays, which was the closing night of the shows at the Apollo and usually slow. In addition there was a competition between four (black) teams from the Savoy and four (white) teams from the Roseland Ballroom. The winner would get a week's work at the Apollo. This was the first time the Savoy dancers would go up against dancers from the Roseland—an irresistible challenge, and it guaranteed that the Savoy dancers would be the best.

All of this meant very little to Sonny and me. We talked it over with our friend Billy and decided maybe we were good enough. We went to the theater to sign up and were told when to report. We practiced every day after school. This was our first contest, and even though we knew we didn't have much of a chance to win, we wanted to look our best.

Since it was the first time the Savoy took on the best dancers from the Roseland, the Savoy group decided to split the prize money—regardless of which of the four black teams won, they would all share the money.

When Sonny and I reported to the theater, we were told to go downstairs to the rehearsal hall in the basement. We were outsiders, and we felt left out of everything. At first no one noticed us, but when they did it was worse, because they snickered amongst themselves. We were just a couple of kids and no one thought we had a chance to win. They seemed a bit irritated that we took one of the four Savoy slots, but not the least bit threatened.

It was in the rehearsal hall that I saw Frank Schiffman for the first time. He ran the theater. He was a very small man who looked like a professor, but he had a lot of power, and he ran a tight ship.

The theater was packed to the rafters and Ralph Cooper was the emcee. "Hey Nacky!" was the by word for the contest; when Coop said it, the house would yell back at him, "Ohhhh Nacky!" This meant the dancers were ready, the audience was ready, and the contest was on.

When it was our turn to dance I was nervous as a cat. We were well rehearsed, and we knew our routine, but we had strong competition. Being kids gave Sonny and me an advantage. The audience was on our side as soon as we swung out. The minute we hit the stage the crowd let out a yell to let us know they were with us. At the time I didn't know it, but my cousin Carlton (who was a teenager himself) was sitting in the front row. He started yelling to me, and Coop picked up on it. He gestured to Carlton to come up on stage. All of this was going on while Sonny and I were dancing. We were so engrossed in our steps that we barely noticed. It wasn't a setup as some of the dancers thought, we didn't even know he was there. Carlton jumped on the stage and started coaching me on; the audience went crazy. The house came down, and we won big that night, the prize money was twenty–five dollars. We left the theater walking on air. Actually it was more like running, because we didn't like the looks we got from the Savoy dancers when we won. We didn't stop running until we got to 132nd Street, across from the Lafayette. Sonny, Billy, and I split the winnings there on the street. We gave Billy five dollars for being our manager, we were each happy with ten dollars.

Our winning that prize created a problem for the Savoy

dancers. Herbert White, their leader, wanted to put the first
Lindy Hop team on stage at the Apollo, but because we
won, we got the week's work. No one knew who we
were or where we had come from, but he was quick to
find out.

The next morning I was getting ready for school when
someone knocked at the door. I ran to the door and asked
who it was. A man's voice told me he was from the theater
where I had danced the night before, and he wanted to talk
to me about my performance.

I opened the door and there were three men. One in
front with two others behind—I later learned that this was
typical Whitey intimidation. Of course, he was charming
and smiling, immediately throwing me off my guard. He
said he was Herbert White. I asked him in and called
Mama, telling her that Mr. White from the theater wanted
to talk to me about my dancing. She said it was all right as
long as it didn't take long, she didn't want me to be late for
school.

Mr. White said he understood that I had to go to school,
and he would just take a minute of my time. He told me
that he thought I was a very good dancer, and he wanted
me to come to the Savoy and dance with his dancers. He
thought I was good enough to dance with them! I was to
come to the Savoy that Saturday and dance under his
direction. Of course I said yes immediately.

I couldn't wait to get to school and tell Sonny. When I
got to school and told him, he wasn't very excited. I was
sure he didn't understand. I felt we could get jobs. We
could be famous. We were invited to dance at the Savoy!
Then Sonny asked if Mr. White had invited him to come

with me. I told him not exactly, but I was sure he meant to and just forgot. We were a team, of course he wanted us both!

At the Savoy on Saturday I learned that friendship came after dancing. Sonny was not asked to join the group. But I was thrilled to be there anyway. Mr. White was there when I arrived and led me to a table near their corner and told me to relax. I sat there watching the group of dancers, barely able to sit still. At last Mr. White pointed someone in my direction, a young man who, eyeing me up and down said, "Let's see what you got kid."

With the first swing–out I began to perform. I knew Mr. White was watching me, and I wanted him to know what I could do. After the second swing–out the dancer abruptly walked me back to my seat, where I stayed for the rest of the evening.

The couples that Sonny and I had defeated in the contest were there. They were good, and it made me proud that we had beat them, but the girls glared at me, and I thought I would never be one of them.

As much as I wanted to get up and dance, I knew I shouldn't. Between the stares of the other dancers and an instant respect for Mr. White, I knew that I shouldn't start dancing on my own.

Mr. White came to me and said,

"How'd you like the show?"

"Show?"

"My dancers! What do ya think I meant? How'd you like it?

"They're fine dancers Mr. White. I'd like to dance with them, I know I'm good enough and . . ."

"Whitey is fine."

"Whitey?"

"My name kid, you can call me Whitey," he said, nearing frustration "you are good. But nobody comes in here and starts dancin' with my kids right away. You got to earn it."

"When you came to my house I thought you asked me to come dance with your dancers and I . . ."

"Look, you ain't even old enough to be in here. If you don't appreciate the invitation, then don't come back."

"N–No sir, Mr., uh, I mean Whitey. I want to come back. I'd come and watch every Saturday if it's okay with you."

"Fine then. It's late, and you should be getting home. I'll see you next Saturday."

Whitey had just taken control of my life, and I hadn't even seen it happen.

The next week Sonny and I were to begin our engagement at the Apollo. It was such an honor to win that we couldn't possibly pass up the opportunity, and there was the twenty–five dollars salary that made it impossible to say no. One tiny problem was that it was an afternoon matinée, and school was still in session. After little debate, Sonny and I agreed to play hooky. It was nearly the end of the school year, and although Sonny and I both loved our classes at P.S. 89, it was an opportunity we couldn't resist.

We were an opening act and the first Lindy Hop team to play the Apollo. Really we were just a couple of kids playing hooky for four days. Having just the two of us on stage looked pretty awful, but we felt we were on our way to fame and fortune! We performed Monday through Thursday, and Friday it was back to school. We each told a

ridiculous tale explaining our absence, and though I doubt
that we were believed, we weren't expelled either.

Saturday it was back to the Savoy and Whitey. No matter
that I wasn't allowed to dance all night, or that I had to
obediently sit and watch. I could not resist the pull of that
beautiful ballroom and the magic of the dance. Dancing
there had been my dream for so long, and at fourteen, I was
inching ever closer to making it come true.

School was soon over, and I was off to camp. Most of the
neighborhood kids scrambled for any summer work, and by
the time I got home from camp the few jobs for kids my
age had long since been taken. I wasn't disappointed
though, I couldn't be bothered with menial labor. I was a
dancer, and dancing was all that I intended to do! Most
afternoons a couple of my girlfriends and I would hang
around the various rehearsal halls. We were always trying to
learn the chorus girls' steps. One particular afternoon we
were hanging around outside of Utopia Hall at 138th Street.
We were on the sidewalk clowning around when without
warning, the door flew open, and out stormed a red–faced
man who looked ready to spit nails. It was the great producer Leonard Reed, whom I recognized. I wondered what
he could possibly be so upset about, but dared not speak to
such an important man.

He looked at the three of us and barked, "Can any of
you dance?"

I said that I danced, we all did. Then he asked us to show
him a time step. We did. Then he asked for an "over the
top" and we did that too. And then, amazingly, he said,
"You're all hired, get in the studio, and let's get going on
this, we haven't much time."

It turned out that Mr. Reed had just fired several of his dancers. Since he had to have his show in Glens Falls in two weeks, he needed replacements, but fast. Oh, the thrill of working for the great Leonard Reed, we couldn't believe that we were hired on the spot!

"We must really be something!" we said as we discussed our careers on the walk home. How thrilled our parents would be that we were going to be real chorus girls. Certainly the small drawback of missing some school would be nothing compared to the respect and recognition we would achieve in the chorus line of Leonard Reed!

We parted ways and went to our homes, and I began to think a little more clearly. Mama would surely wring my neck if I told her I wanted to return to school late—or possibly not at all to travel with a chorus line. I knew she wouldn't hear of it, but if I went to all the rehearsals and then told her right before we left for the trip, she couldn't say no.

The next day I reported to Utopia Hall for rehearsal. Only one of my friends was waiting outside for me and she was looking down in the mouth. When I asked her what was up, she told me that her mama and daddy wouldn't let her go. They said that Mr. Reed had no business putting young girls in his chorus line, and her daddy nearly came down here to tell him so himself.

When I asked her where our third chorus girl was, she said she couldn't come either and that her mama gave her a beating for even hanging around down there. She wasn't going to be allowed to come out with us until school started.

Then she asked me what Mama had said about my

joining the group. I stretched the truth a little and said "Oh, you know Mama, she's always supportive of my dancin'." Then I told her I'd see her when I saw her. My main concern was that their quitting didn't ruin my own chances. It didn't.

The two weeks of rehearsal went well. I was put in the back line, but I picked up the steps quickly and easily. The time also went quickly, and before I knew it, it was the first week of school. I had to tell Mama I had other plans. She was furious! I begged, I cried, I pleaded.

Mama finally threw her hands in the air and said, "Fine! You go, but if the truant officers come looking for you I'm not gonna lie to 'em, and if they want to come and throw your skinny little ass in jail I'll let 'em!"

It was settled, I left for Glens Falls and my big career as a chorus girl. Less than a week later, while running through a rehearsal at the theater, a man came in asking questions. I could see him from the stage and thought nothing of it. But before I knew it, Mr. Reed was standing at the foot of the stage, with the man shouting, "Miss Miller, could you be so kind as to join us for a moment?"

I walked off the stage and joined them. Mr. Reed's face was red, and I knew I was in for it. The strange man spoke up and asked if my name was Norma Miller, daughter of Alma Miller, residing in Harlem? Nervously I said that it was and asked what the problem was. He told me that the problem was that I belonged in school not in a theater.

I looked at Mr. Reed, and he simply shook his head and walked off. I knew I had no choice but to go with the officer and wait for my mother.

After several days waiting in the detention center and a miserable train ride home with Mama, I returned to P.S. 89

and to my friends and my normal teenage life. I also returned to the Savoy on Saturdays. I nearly didn't get in the
first week back, but one of Whitey's dancers, Frankie
Manning spotted me and talked Big George into letting me
in. "Where you been kid? Whitey was askin' if anyone had
seen you."

"I've been real busy with school" I lied.

I had no intention of letting Whitey in on my chorus
experience. Partially out of embarrassment, but mostly
because I had a strange sense of loyalty to him. The other
dancers warmed to me, and I began to get out on the floor.
Whitey didn't seem to mind, he appeared to enjoy watching me dance.

Poverty continued to flourish in Harlem, and though I
lived in the middle of it, I was able to overlook it. I loved
my classes at P.S. 89, and every weekend I fell into the
fantasy world of the Savoy. I was blind to the frustration
and anger building in my own neighborhood, but in March
1935 the rage exploded and could no longer be ignored.[1]

A young Puerto Rican boy had been caught stealing in a
five and dime store. It was said that the manager, who was a
white man, caught him and beat him. The story spread
throughout the community like wild fire. This, combined
with the frustrations of a people living in poverty and being
discriminated against in their own community ignited a riot.
The riot resulted in four deaths, many injuries, and hundreds of thousands of dollars in damage.[2]

[1] Hamilton, Charles V., *The Political Biography of an American
Dilemma: Adam Clayton Powell, Jr.* (New York: Atheneum, 1991), 56.
[2] Ibid.

Harlem was crying out, and once again, Adam Clayton Powell, Jr., responded. At first he could not understand why the people of Harlem would destroy their own community. Surely they could see that this would only worsen their living conditions. But as he looked further he saw the black community's anger stemmed from the fact that although they lived there, Harlem was owned by the whites. They weren't even being employed in the stores in which they spent what little money they had. When Powell took a survey of nearly five thousand people working on 125th Street, he found that only ninety–three of them were black, and all were doing menial labor.[3] There was not one black cashier or manager. Within days after the riot, Powell had organized the Coordinating Committee for Employment.[4] Using the slogan, "Don't buy where you can't work" the committee organized picket lines in front of stores up and down 125th Street. Eventually this discrimination ended.

After the riot, Mayor La Guardia made desperate appeals for calm. In his effort to restore peace he asked all merchants to post the following leaflet in their windows:

Malice and viciousness of the instigators are betrayed by the false statements in mimeographed hand bills and placards. Attempts may be made to repeat the spreading of false gossip of misrepresentation in hand bills or other printed matter. I appeal to the law abiding element of Harlem to carefully scrutinize any charge, rumor, or gossip of racial discrimination being made at this time. Every agency of the city is available to assist in investigating all such charges. I expect a complete

[3] Haskins, 36.
[4] Ibid.

report giving me details of everything that occurred. As soon as I receive these reports they will be made public.[5]

The Savoy was damaged in the riot and closed to repair the damage. This caused further discontent and concern within the community.

Even Adam Clayton Powell, Jr., was disturbed. As the only totally integrated place in New York, the Savoy hired black people in all capacities. Powell also loved the music and the dancing, he was as suited for the dance floor on Saturday as he was for the pulpit on Sunday. He felt the Savoy was far too important a place to be closed for any length of time, especially in these tense times.

A meeting was called between Savoy owner Moe Gale, manager Charlie Buchanan, and Whitey to discuss what could be done about the damaged property and the community's damaged morale. Something needed to be done, to raise Harlem's tattered spirits and to restore the ballroom's business.

Whitey, Mr. Buchanan, and two men from the *Daily News* met to discuss a dance contest that the paper wanted to sponsor as their contribution to boosting morale after the riot.

Whitey was introduced as the prime motivation behind the dancing seen at the ballroom. Recognizing the popularity of the Lindy Hop the newspaper men wanted the Savoy in a competition that would pit dancers from all the boroughs against one another in one event. This wouldn't be just a local contest, they wanted it to be city–wide and to include the Waltz, the Fox Trot, the Rhumba, the Tango,

[5] Hamilton, 57.

and the Lindy. They felt it would be good exposure for everyone involved—inlcuding the *Daily News*.

Whitey agreed that it sounded like a great idea, but he was concerned. The Lindy Hop was a dance that had broken away from traditional dance aesthetics. Though we loved competition, he didn't know if we could compete in all categories, and was concerned that judges who didn't know the Lindy would be using inappropriate standards.

Mr. Buchanan agreed with Whitey. Nonetheless everyone knew that no one in any of the five boroughs could out–dance the kids from the Savoy in the Lindy. The rules would simply have to be adjusted. The Savoy probably couldn't take the all around championship with the Lindy Hop, but it could sure get a lot of attention. It was the most popular dance out there. The Savoy had to participate, it wouldn't be a contest without the Savoy involved. Whitey agreed to participate only if his kids had a clean shot at the Lindy.

When Whitey left the meeting he called Frankie Manning and Leon James over to discuss the contest; they were his two main dancers, and he always told them his plans before the rest of us. They sat in a booth deep in conversation, but we couldn't hear what it was about.

Later when we learned about the contest we were told that it was our chance to put the Lindy on the map, and we needed to start rehearsing yesterday. Whitey told us that we would meet at the ballroom daily and work out the routines. He had to decide who was going to dance for us and get anybody who didn't have a regular partner someone to work with. He figured it would be an elimination contest, and the best of the lot would compete in the finals. He let us know that this was it! We were gonna let the world know about the Lindy and that it belonged to us!

Whitey was the leader, and we obeyed. He paired me up with Billy Hill, "Stompin' Billy" as we called him. He was a good dancer, and I didn't mind a bit. The contest was called the Harvest Moon Ball, and rehearsing for it became the main focus of our lives.

A MAN CALLED WHITEY

In the spring of 1927, while the rest of the country was still debating the morals of the Charleston, a new step in the evolution of dance had begun in Harlem. The new dance, at first called simply the Hop, was pioneered by dancers like Shorty Snowden, a small man of five feet, two inches who danced a comedy act with his partner, Big Bea who was a towering six feet, and George "Twist Mouth" Ganaway.

In May, Charles Lindbergh became a folk hero when he made the world's first solo flight across the Atlantic by taking off from a New York airport and landing in Paris. Because of the new dance's own delightful "solo hops" the dance was called the Lindy Hop.

Herbert White, known as Whitey or Mac, was immediately attracted to it and decided to capitalize on the new dance. The Lindy was far more exciting than any of the other dances floating around Harlem and suited the letter and the spirit of jazz perfectly. Two eight–count Lindy steps matched up with one four measure jazz phrase, both involved the repetition of basic patterns that were never executed the same way twice. The Lindy, therefore, could evolve with the music.

The Shorty Snowden Trio was the first professional team to take the dance outside the ballroom. The trio was actually three teams; the first was Shorty and Big Bea. The second couple, the mighty Leroy (Stretch) and his petite dancing partner Little Bea were fast and smooth as silk, they always broke it up when they swung out. Rounding up the trio was a brother and sister team, Madeline and Freddie. The Lindy was also performed by Twist Mouth George who was number one in the ballroom. He and his partner worked alone, and when Twist Mouth swung out, the house came down. It was the work of these teams around the city that showed Whitey the potential of the dance. So he tried to organize these dancers. He offered to manage them and handle their dates. He promised them higher pay and better working conditions. But, he couldn't convince them that being under one umbrella would improve their bookings and extend the life of the new dance craze. As the opportunities increased it became more and more apparent to these veteran dancers that Whitey was trying to monopolize the dance. This led to an internal struggle in the ballroom and Whitey's decision to find his own dancers and form his own group.

By the early 1930s he had become the floor manager at the Savoy, and he used his position and his knowledge of the dance to full advantage. He knew just the kind of dancers he was looking for; they had to be young, stylized, and, most of all, they had to have a beat, they had to swing. He would walk amongst them, always smiling and charming. You could easily recognize him by the two–inch white streak that parted his hair in the center, his well developed body over a stocky frame, a complexion that looked like a Hawaiian tan, and smiling brown eyes that crinkled at the edges. He had a full bottom lip that would instantly give his

"They played the Cotton Club in 1938 and then joined the Eugene Howard Review and went to Australia."

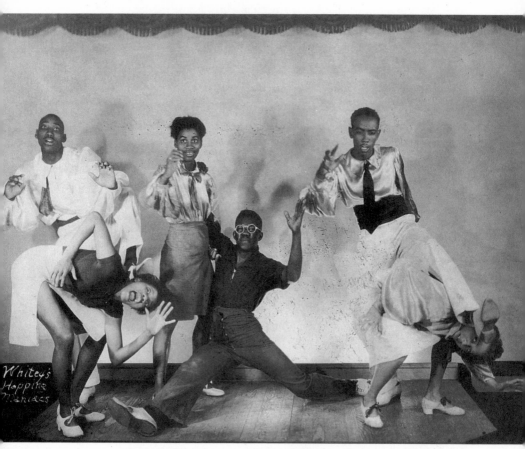

Whitey's Hopping Maniacs, Frank Manning and Naomi Wallace, Lucille Middleton and Jerome, Billy Williams and Millie (left to right), later to become known as Whitey's Lindy Hoppers, performing at the Cotton Club.

mood away. If he was displeased it trembled; when he was happy it broke into a wide grin.

He was street wise and he knew young people, he knew how to motivate them. He knew his dance and selected his dancers carefully. When he saw dancers with potential, he set out to get them in his group. Prowling the dance floor he would encourage the dancers as he sized them up, looking only for the best. He invited the dancers with great potential over to the northeast (141st Street) corner of the ballroom, just to the right of the band shell. There he would train them, molding them into a faithful member of his group.

Working in the ballroom gave Whitey an additional advantage. Whenever a call came in requesting dancers, Whitey was the one who supplied them. All of the shows being packaged from the ballroom included Lindy Hoppers, and Whitey was booking his own dancers for these jobs. And so he began building his dancing dynasty. From the beginning Whitey had a clear view of his goal. He wanted to be the man to make the Lindy Hop a famous and accepted art form—he was to be the Balanchine of the Lindy Hoppers. He wanted new dancers who would start where the old ones left off. He would show those fools that if they didn't get together and get a base pay for trios, doubles, and singles, they would be nowhere. Getting jobs without proper representation made no sense to him. Within a few years he had his own talented collection of kids and was ready to challenge Shorty Snowden, Twist Mouth, and the others; he wanted to be crowned King of the Lindy Hop.

Whitey's two main dancers were Leon James and Frank Manning. Leon was a holdover from Whitey's days as a club organizer and dancer. Leon was a flashy dancer who could steal a scene with his bugging eyes and wiggly knees. He would constantly point his finger at his partner with a steady beat. Despite the widely recognized fact that Leon was one of the top dancers in the ballroom, it was always said that Whitey inherited Leon, but he picked Frankie. Whitey loved Frankie. You could see it in his eyes as he watched him dance—the love of a proud father. Frankie represented everything that was best in Lindy Hop dancing. He could execute, swing, lift a girl effortlessly, and never miss a beat. It was with Frankie that Whitey began the first of the ensemble dancing that moved the Lindy Hop from a dance in a ballroom to a slick professional act that became a show stopper in theaters around the country.

Whitey had spotted Frankie dancing in the center of the Savoy ballroom; not yet daring to join the superior dancers on the 141st side. Frankie was with a date as well as Billy and Willamae Ricker. They usually danced at the Renaissance Ballroom for the under twenty–one year–olds and were a bit intimidated by the Savoy. Frankie was shocked when Whitey approached him.

Whitey politely interrupted their conversation and asked Frankie if he would come over to the corner for a minute and meet some of his dancers. Frankie accepted for the whole group, but Whitey quickly excluded the others. Frankie told Whitey he would prefer to stay with his friends.

Whitey left, but Frankie could see him still watching from the other side of the ballroom. Frankie began throwing in special little moves just to get a reaction. After several visits to the Savoy, Whitey gave in and invited Frankie's friends to come along with him to his side of the ballroom. So began an association that would last a very long time.[1]

The Lindy Hoppers were in great demand in the ballroom. Every night you could see Whitey walking amongst his dancers, coaching them. He looked like a football coach on the sidelines; pacing up and down, leading the cheering section, and applauding whenever a dancer did a step that delighted the patrons. When the tourists came to the ballroom, they saw what they thought was a spontaneous exhibition by a regular group of dancers, simply in a ballroom to enjoy social dancing. But that wasn't the case, what they were watching was rehearsed and choreographed dance. Whitey was the original stage mother, he left nothing to chance. Every detail was worked out in advance, and when the visitors came, he was ready for them. With a nod of his head, or a gesture, Whitey would send a dancer out on the floor. They moved to his beat, and with the best bands in the country to practice with, getting results was never a problem.

Whitey, the guru of Swing, the man who was determined to take the Lindy around the world, appeared to be as completely devoted to his dancers as they were to him. Some had reason to be skeptical. Take William Downes for instance. He and his sister Joyce had begun dancing the Lindy Hop at a very young age. At first they would only go to the Renaissance for Sunday matinées. Eventually they began branching out, testing their skills in other ballrooms, and began to get work in various shows in places like the Harlem Opera House and the Lafayette Theater. At twelve and thirteen years old, they were each being paid seventy–

[1] Frank Manning, dancer, personal interview, 1984.

five dollars a week. William and Joyce were such a hit that they were held over for three weeks at the Lafayette. They were making money, were booking performances themselves, and didn't feel they needed an agent. They managed to become a popular dance team around Harlem without one. William had even been handed the Lindy Hop crown by Twist Mouth George, also known as Susquehanna, himself. Twist Mouth even called William Young Susque. They did have a lot in common: they swung out the same way, and when they entered the floor dancing, the crowds would yell, loving their every move.

William had heard rumors that Whitey wanted him and Joyce to join the Lindy Hoppers. He didn't think much of it, because he felt he and his sister were doing fine on their own. One day though, Whitey approached William, accompanied by his goons, the Jolly Fellows as they were called, and young William was instantly intimidated. Then Whitey got nasty telling him that if he didn't dance with the group he would not be allowed to dance at the Savoy. William was shaken and agreed to join Whitey's group.

Whitey was the main man in the ballroom and everyone did their best to please him. As much as the older dancers tried to talk the kids out of Whitey's direction, they remained loyal to him. Whitey's dancers all believed that the older set was simply jealous of their youth and refused to hear the warnings. William, however, felt going with Whitey meant a big salary cut, and he certainly never got a share of the suitcases full of money he saw Whitey with.[2]

There were definitely two sides to Whitey.

[2] William Downes, dancer, personal interview, 1982.

THE HARVEST MOON BALL

The *Daily News'* Harvest Moon Ball was hailed as the world's greatest dancing contest for ballroom dancing. It would be the Olympics of the dancing world, a pantathlon of events—the Waltz, Tango, Rhumba, Fox Trot, and the Lindy Hop. Contests were held in all five of the boroughs, with the winners competing in a grand finals to determine the all around champions. It was the popularity of the Lindy Hop that inspired the contest, but it was the one dance that didn't fit the rules of ballroom dancing. All of the other categories had the same standards: elegance, smoothness, grace, and fluid lines. Partners were always to touch each other and their feet had to remain on the floor at all times. None of these applied to the Lindy Hop; it seemed out of place in an elegant setting. Its moves would be hidden or impossible in the white tie and tails and beautiful ball gowns worn by the other dancers. Lindy Hop dancers wore flat shoes with rubber soles to grip the floor and the women's skirts were usually very short to allow for freer movement.

At the time the Fox Trot and Waltz, traditional ballroom dances which had been danced for years, were executed with very little variety. The Tango and Rhumba differed in rhythm but still looked the same in their presentations. The steps were set down in patterns that hadn't changed in years. The way the couple moved together, the way the women held their dresses, and the turn of the head was prescribed. They were beautiful and graceful, but like paper dolls that moved and stepped in unison. What varied was the degree of smoothness and grace each couple achieved. But the Lindy defied the judges' imaginations. The music was faster than any music ever played in a contest. The couple's attire was more like sports attire. The steps had not been danced on a ballroom floor before; although the dancers were not as acrobatic as they would later become, they still were faster and flashier than any of the other contestants. The judges had to have their eyes wide open. No two teams would dance alike, and the advantage would go to the one who first captured the judge's eye. The dancers who were the best in Lindy contests knew how to play for the judge's eye because they were used to being on display.

Preparing for the Harvest Moon Ball consumed all of our time. We were all a bit apprehensive about it, because for the first time we were to be judged by people outside our own audience. We were dancers used to being crowd pleasers, but not accustomed to being given rules such as those that the dance committee was setting down for us. It bothered us that we had no point of reference. The only judges we had performed for were the audiences themselves. If they liked you, you won. That was all there was to it. Now we were going to be judged on a point system. There were points for grace, execution, originality, and appearance. And everyone looked to the Savoy to bring in the top Lindy Hop dancers.

Of course there were the standard ballroom dancers who signed up, but Whitey's main concern was the Lindy Hoppers. He wanted the Lindy Hop crown, he felt the other ballrooms could have all the other champions, but the Lindy Hop was his—the crown had to be won for the Savoy.

The night of the semi-finals, the Savoy was packed to the rafters. The entire staff was decked out in tuxedos and gowns. Tonight the Savoy was playing host to the New York press, and it was always good business to impress the press. Charlie Buchanan and his entire staff were on their toes.

The dancers were told to be at the ballroom early, so as not to be lost in the large crowd that had gathered to see the contest. We were assembled at the far end of the ball-room, the 140th Street side, to line up for the grand march. There were quite a number of contestants for this first Harvest Moon Ball. There were more Lindy Hop teams than ballroom teams, but the number of ballroom dancers was still impressive. The Sheik's was the ballroom team that stood out. Despite his odd appearance, he was an excep-tional ballroom dancer and the one to watch in the Fox Trot and the Tango. The Sheik was a fair skinned black man wearing a white suit with large lapels, and his hair was slicked down Rudolph Valentino style. His moustache was waxed and curled up at the ends. His dancing partner was wearing a long red gown and she had a rose in her hair, looking very Spanish in style. Despite the contrast between the Sheik and the Lindy Hoppers, he was a good contestant and a favorite of ours.

The music struck and the Grand March began. Jack Larue and his staff led the march across the dance floor, and the audience and judges saw the contestants for the first time. The house cheered as the Lindy Hoppers took the floor, it was bound to be a big night.

The atmosphere in the ballroom was electric. The Savoy looked like a palace. The chandeliers shone like giant stars, brilliant in the dark night. The deep red pile carpet seemed to have grown, and you sunk down into it as you walked. Everyone looked radiant, especially Whitey. He was beaming as bright as a star himself. He looked great in his tux, and his white streak was as white as snow; tonight, everything about him glowed. He was realizing a dream, his dancers were the ones to watch tonight. This would bring him to the attention of the press, precisely what he needed to bring his dancers before the public. For weeks the press had been hyping the contest and saying, look out for the Lindy Hoppers at the Savoy. It was this that gave Whitey his extra edge. He knew it was his Lindy Hoppers who brought the excitement to the contest.

All the dances in the ballroom had their roots in a foreign country, but the Lindy Hop was created in New York. In Harlem. At the Savoy. It was an American dance created by Americans. It had soul, and it had swing, which is what made it popular everywhere it was introduced.

The contest began, the first dance was the Fox Trot. As usual, it was graceful, very elegant, and smooth. A marvelous exhibition of two people tuned in to one another. The Sheik and his partner performed beautifully, but it was when the Sheik danced the Tango that he stole the judges' hearts. The entire audience applauded, and as hoped, he was the dancer to represent the Savoy in the finals.

The Lindy Hop dominated the contest at the Savoy, it was what everyone was waiting for. It began with Charlie Buchanan announcing, "And now, the Lindy Hop." The house let out a howl. Instead of dancing one team at a time as was usual, we danced four teams at a time. That meant the judges had to shift their attention between dancers. It was like watching a four-ring circus. We knew that the winner would be the first to attract the judges' attention. We were a group of dancers used to stealing that extra bow, our instincts served us well.

The contest was held in front of the band shell. The band on the stage was the mighty Chick Webb Band and this was what they had been waiting for. Here the music would swing, at last they could pull out the stops and let it rip. No one could push a band quite like Chick Webb could, he had what was called a kicking-the-ass-beat. The Lindy Hop was developed to his music. The first swing-out was like madness. It was every man for himself. The loud yell from the dancers meant that it was on. They made noises similar to those of martial arts, the sound that releases pent-up energy.

Leon James and Edith Mathews, Frank Manning and Maggie McMillian, William and Sarah Downes, and Billy Hill and I were expected to win. We lived up to Whitey's expectations; the audience and the judges were thrilled with our display of swinging jazz dancing. Chick Webb's band played like they never had before, and the whole place was swinging. This didn't mean that the other ballroom dancers were not important, for they were, and they gave beautiful presentations of the traditional ballroom dances. The traditional dance teams simply did not create the interest that the Lindy Hoppers created.

The final judgment was predictable. All the teams were picked to go to the finals. The judges couldn't pick one team over another, so they chose us all. I guess they wanted to be sure and get out of Harlem without any trouble—if you know what I mean. The top winners in the contest were Leon and Edith, Frankie and Maggie, and Billy and me. The Sheik and his partner and all of the Lindy Hop teams were going to the finals; the Savoy would be well represented.

To see our reactions, you would think we had won a million dollars instead of a contest, but it was an important contest. We were in the dancing business, and a competition like the Harvest Moon Ball was good for the ballroom and everyone involved.

The elation seemed to rub off on everyone, from the girl downstairs in the cloakroom to the top ballroom managers, Moe Gale and Charles Buchanan; to see Charlie Buchanan smile, you knew it was a good night.

After the contest Whitey met with our group of dancers and gave us our instructions for the next day. Now there was no grumbling about being in the ballroom for rehearsals. We were all so excited. Whitey could have asked us to do anything, and we would have broken our necks to do it.

The next day the papers were full of the contest. The photographers had captured it, and they printed photographs of the dancers. We were gathered at the Savoy reading the paper. There was Leon, grinning like a Cheshire cat. He had really come through, he'd had the audience screaming with his antics. He was a good Lindy Hopper, but his real talent was blinding the judges with his flash, and it worked. Leon's partner Edith Mathews was fast. She had created the Lindy step; she had a sit down twist that made her whole body look like a pretzel. Her dance style was different; she was from the Charleston era and had the look

of a Swing girl of her time. Anywhere she danced she
would bring out her whole neighborhood. They were her
rooting section, and whenever they announced the names,
"Leon and Edith" you would hear the roar and know that
she had her fan club with her.

We all knew that Frankie was the best dancer. It was
Frankie's dancing that most dancers wanted to imitate. His
partner for this contest was his size, which didn't balance
well for his kind of dancing. Frankie always danced well
with any partner, but with the right partner he was
matchless.

Whitey was hoping that Frankie and Leon would walk
away with the top prize. He knew that a champion would
be in demand to perform. He planned to team the two of
them and get bookings on the strength of their champion-
ships. With his access to the ballroom bookings, he knew he
would have an easy sell to clubs and theaters across the
country, but first, they had to win.

Whitey told the rest of us to keep up our routines, that
he would check in on us and keep us informed of any
contest details as he got them. Meanwhile, he turned his
attention to Leon and Frankie. He knew they'd make a
dynamite team, but he wanted to be safe. He took them to
the upstairs Apollo rehearsal hall, which would be their's
until after the contest. With the championship in his hands,
he would be ready for his dancers to take over where the
Shorty Snowden group had left off.

It wasn't required that we be in the ballroom everyday.
We were more or less a back-up group, but we had all
become like family, and it was difficult to stay away. My
partner, Stompin' Billy, and I had become especially good

friends. There was no romance involved—Whitey strictly forbade romance between dancing partners—but we just loved clowning around together. It kept the fun in rehearsing.

The Harvest Moon Ball finals were going to be held at the Central Park Mall. It was going to be a festive night, dancing under the stars, the harvest moon! What could be more appropriate? It was announced that the ball music would be played by the Abe Lyman Orchestra and, for the Lindy Hop, the great Fletcher Henderson Orchestra. There would be a band shell for the two orchestras, and they were going to erect a dance floor. The audience would gather all around the dance floor. All plans were in place for a wonderful evening of dancing and, hopefully, victory.

On the night of the finals we were told to meet in the ballroom to get our instructions by five P.M. and to come prepared to stay until it was all over. We were to bring our clothes with us, as we wouldn't be able to return home before the contest. We would be taken to dinner, then driven to the park by bus and deposited backstage.

We all assembled in the ballroom before five and typically, we were horsing around.

The anticipation began to overwhelm us as the time approached. We joined all the other contestants for dinner, and though everyone was smiling and seemed happy, there was a natural nervousness that accompanies competition. All of the contestants were white except for the teams from the Savoy. There were twelve of our teams in all, and it was an eerie feeling when we entered the dining room en mass. Surprisingly, the atmosphere was natural, happy, and we fell right in as if we had known each other forever. We were assured of our place in the contest; we knew there was nothing to worry about from the other contestants. We had this one wrapped up, no one could come up against a Savoy Lindy Hopper and win, we would make sure of this. Tonight, the Lindy Hop was represented by the top teams of the Savoy.

While we were having dinner we heard that the place was jammed, there was a huge crowd; more people had shown up than had been anticipated. We were getting the news in bits and pieces as we prepared to board the buses taking us to the event.

On the bus taking us from dinner to the park, the entire group joined in a sing-along. It was a glorious night, perfect for dancing. The bus was unable to enter the park where planned because there were people everywhere, and we couldn't get through. The driver tried another entrance, but still we couldn't get in. We were all calling out, "Hey let us in! There can't be a contest without contestants! Get out of the way!" All we could see were people everywhere. It was a mob out of control, and we couldn't get in.

After all the preparations, the anxiety, the pent-up emotions, the contest was called off to protect the safety of the public. It was to be rescheduled for a later date when it could be better organized.

We were taken back to the Savoy, drained of emotions. We talked nonsense to cover up our disappointment and gathered at the Savoy. Some of us stayed and danced the night away. I went off to camp.

I didn't know it at the time, but the summer of 1935 was to be an important one for me. Just like every summer before, Mama had made arrangements to get us on the list for camp. And just like every summer before, I went off to camp in Connecticut, a recipient of some wealthy woman's generosity, someone who had donated her property so that the poor Harlem kids could spend a couple of weeks away from the hot city. This summer was to be the same, I thought, and to camp I went. I was very disappointed and glad to be getting away. I couldn't help but wonder about the contest. How would it have come out? Who would have won? I believed that Billy and I could have won.

On August 23, we were all going about our regular activities, when I noticed a small mob had gathered around a picnic table. A couple of the older girls in the crowd were yelling out to me, "Hey Norma, c'mere you're in the newspaper!"

I ignored them because I didn't believe them. So they came to me, newspaper in hand, and showed me. The headline read "Dance Thrill Awaits 18,500 at Garden." The article said:

All kinds of dancing—dreamy Waltzes, smooth Fox Trots and swash-buckling Tangos to twisting Rhumbas and snappy Lindy Hops will be done to perfection by the finest amateur dancers in the metropolitan area Wednesday night at the finals of the *Daily News* Harvest Moon Ball at Madison Square Garden.

No matter how you like your dancing, you'll be thrilled by the performances of the eighty-two couples who've come through the eliminations to battle before 18,500 spectators for the terpsichorean crowns awaiting the winners.

The article went on to mention the Lindy Hop contest.

Just before the last event of the night goes on, the contest for the all-around championship, you'll see the finals of the Lindy Hop.

When Fletcher Henderson and his orchestra, the smoothest aggregation of colored musicians in town, start playing for the Lindy Hoppers you'll see action.

And then astoundingly, they mentioned me!

We don't remember all of the 82 couples individually, but we'll never forget the stepping of a few of them. There's Norma Miller and Bill Hill as a starter. Norma and Bill are two of Harlem's favorites, a couple of youngsters who were born with syncopation in their veins, with a strutting in their nature.

Then there's Frank Manning and Maggie McMillian. They're from Harlem too, and when they get on the floor at the garden your eyes will dart from Bill and Norma to Frank and Maggie.[1]

All my friends started talking at once. "You've got to go back, they think you can win!" I was just flabbergasted. Me. They were talking about my dancing, and I couldn't believe it. Yet, there it was in black and white. I ran to the administration office as fast as I could. I burst into the office, talking and stammering and waving the article. I must have looked like I had a good case of hysterics because the counselor tried to calm me down. First she made me sit down and take a deep breath, and then, asked me for the story. I showed her the article in the paper, and she too got excited. Everyone in the camp knew that I was going to be a dancer, and the fact that one of their charges attracted such attention was a feather in their hat.

There was no doubt about it, I had to go back immediately.

[1] Turcott, Jack. "Dance Thrill Awaits 18,500 at Garden." *New York Daily News*, August 23, 1935.

Mama and Dot agreed. Although Mama had never approved of my affiliation with the Lindy—she had hoped I would pursue a more "respectable" dance career—her smile told me that she was proud of me. They immediately began to process me out of camp and arranged for my transportation back to New York. Before I could say "jack rabbit," I was getting ready to go to the train heading home, my head full of wild dreams.

I said my goodbyes to all my camp gang, not knowing when I would ever see them again. We had spent so much of our lives together each summer, and as I left in the pick-up truck for the train, I was both melancholy and exhilarated. Part of my life was ending and another world was opening up for me.

By the time the train pulled out of the Milford, Connecticut station, I could think of nothing but what a great dance contest this was going to be. And now, it was going to be at Madison Square Garden! When I got back to New York I raced for the Savoy.

When I arrived, Whitey kissed me on the cheek and said, "Hey Sweetie, glad you're back. I was wondering if you were going to make the big contest."

I told him that after the fiasco at the mall, I wasn't sure there was going to be a contest. I showed him the article and he beamed, "Yeah, looks great don't it? And you thought I was ignoring you, didn't you? Listen, I never worry where your dancing is concerned, I know you're going to do great things. You're one of my prize dancers, you know that don't you?"

It was the first time he had ever said anything like that to me. I looked at him and all I could say was, "Thanks Mac." But I knew that he and I had reached a new understanding. I knew that everything was going to be all right.

The next happy face I ran into was my partner Billy Hill's, he was excited to see me and wondered how I'd found out about the contest. I told him it was big news— even in Connecticut.

He grabbed my arm and dragged me to the corner. Lowering his voice he told me that he was excited about more than my being back for the contest. He had found a girl, and her name was Melissa, he said she was beautiful.

When I asked if I knew her and if she danced, he said she wasn't from uptown, but that dancing was how he'd met her. She had come in with a girlfriend on a Sunday, and she wanted lessons, he had been seeing her ever since. Then he told me Whitey wasn't too happy about it and that she was on her way over. He wanted me to cover for him.

"Damn Billy, a big contest about ready to go on and you've got time for girls?" I asked jokingly. "Really, I don't blame Whitey. You should be spending your time practicing, not giving lessons. No wonder he's hot with you."

Billy said that Whitey wasn't so much upset with how he was spending his time as he was with who he was spending it with.

I asked him, "What, is this Melissa so beautiful that he wants her too?"

Before he could answer, his eyes shot to the entrance, and he told me she was there. He begged me to distract Whitey just long enough for him to leave. I couldn't turn him down.

"All right Billy," I said, "but be back soon, we need to get working if we're gonna pull this mother off!"

He thanked me and bolted toward the entrance. I followed him with my eyes, I had to see this girl and what all of the fuss was about. When I saw who he walked up to, my jaw dropped. She was beautiful all right. Beautiful and lily white, with long red hair. No wonder Whitey was upset. That was the last worry he needed with so much already going on.

I made my rounds saying hello to everyone and getting back in the swing of things, waiting for Billy to get back. When he did, I let him have it. "What are you thinkin' about, running around with a white girl like that? She looks like a rich one too. Don't you know that's exactly the kind of thing got people wanting to close us down?"

Billy looked shocked by my reaction, reminding me nobody cared about that at the Savoy, that white girls was always dancing with the black fellers. It's the way the Savoy was. He said they just liked each other, so they were spendin' some time together. Nobody was gettin' hurt.

I felt he was heading for trouble but we didn't have time to argue. I told him I hoped he knew what he was getting into, and we started dancing.

More rehearsals, more steps. The day finally came to go to the Garden. Whitey met us in the ballroom so as to be sure there would be no stragglers. He was a stickler for time and always made sure his group was punctual. He gave us the regular pep talk before we left. He sat on the floor with us around him, campfire style. I sat near him, right at his feet, and sitting there, I felt like I was his kid and he was the father I never had.

"Tonight," he said, "you're going up against real competition. We've got to show them what the Lindy Hop is all about. That we are the champs. You have got to bring back that championship. You are the flag bearers of the Savoy, and you know what we expect you to do tonight. Go out there and let 'em know who we are. Let the *Daily News* report that we took it all, first, second, and third! We want all three. Remember, we don't take out any other prizes. All we got is the Lindy Hop so you better make sure it belongs to us. Do you dig?"

"We dig!" we all said at once.

He knew how to fire us up. Whitey had a way of instilling pride in us and making us want to go out there and do it, and we knew we could. Whitey knew how to get into the heart and soul of the dancers.

When we arrived at the Garden, we were led, in line, to the arena. There we would mount the steps to the central platform that was to be the dance floor.

We rehearsed our routines from top to bottom, and then the music began for the parade of dancers. Our hearts were pounding. We entered the garden to the music of Abe Lyman. Four teams at a time would be competing. The maestro and the head of the contest had told us that we would parade around the floor and then sit around the dance floor but continue to move up musical-chairs style as one team finished and another began. We were the last team before the all-around champions were to dance.

I saw Whitey come into the Garden. He was there to give us moral support and last minute instructions. He had no official job with the contest, but he was welcomed as the boss from the Savoy.

As we watched the rehearsals for the Fox Trot, Billy and I were straining our eyes, searching the gathering crowd for familiar faces. I knew Billy was looking for Melissa, and I hoped that she would come, I knew it was important to him. Finally it was our turn and then the rehearsal ended. We were led back two by two and were told that we would go to dinner, after which we would return to the Garden for the final event.

At dinner we were introduced to the other dancers. They were from all professions. There were waiters, porters, doormen, secretaries, hairdressers; anyone who loved dancing. Some people danced only on their nights off, while others were looking for a professional career. Some would reach glorious heights and others would fall back into oblivion. Whitey in particular, saw this as a mile stone. He saw in this contest a future for the Lindy Hop.

The contest began at eight P.M., sharp. We lined up for the Grand March—it was a sight to see. The women wore ball gowns and were gorgeous. The men wore tails and white ties. The only thing that looked out of place was the huge identifying number that the men wore on their coats, making them look like walking billboards. As the first of the teams entered the arena, we could hear the reaction of the audience. They wanted to see a great dance contest, and they would not be disappointed.

The noise increased as the Lindy Hoppers, the last in line, entered. We could hear the audience was with us, and we responded to their yells by swinging when we walked. Harlem was on parade. All taboos were broken when it came to the Lindy.

The emcee was Milton Berle, who introduced the first ballroom dancers. We were privileged to see the dancing De Marcos, who were the top dance team of the day, they were polished and exquisite.

The women were lovely with their gowns sweeping the floor. Their hair was pulled up in buns at the napes of their necks so as to show a clear line from the base of the neck to their spines, which were held with great dignity. Some of the men were stevedores, carpenters, and janitors, wearing white tie and tails for the first time in their lives. Some looked as if they were born for that attire. Most of the contestants held low-income jobs, dancing was their way of escaping. Then the maestro raised his baton and gave the down beat. The first Harvest Moon Ball began.

As the competition started, the contestants began their circular progression around the dance floor, a magnificent sight. The music was "Shine on, Harvest Moon," the theme of the contest. The first competition was in the Fox Trot, with four teams dancing at one time. Even we got caught up in the contest, as the first winners were announced and yelps of joy went up for them. When the time came for the Lindy competition, the yell from the crowd could be heard all the way back to Harlem. Here the great Fletcher Henderson took over, and the first of the Lindy Hoppers hit the stage. These were the white Lindy Hoppers from the outer areas of New York. They seemed clumsy to us. Watching them butcher our dance made our tempers flare, and this made us even more determined to take the crown home. After the last of the white Lindy Hoppers left, Harlem came on. By this time we were like a group of caged animals, ready to burst from the box. Fletcher Henderson raised his baton, and thus began the wildest dance exhibition that had ever been seen.

The Savoy Lindy Hoppers took first, second, and third prizes. Whitey was beaming, he had won it all. His dancers had taken it, just as he'd predicted. He had no stake in any of the other dances, which was why his dancers had to sweep their category. The house went wild when they announced the winners. Leon and Edith were dancing in each others arms, and Frankie and Maggie were laughing and crying. I jumped up when they called my name and dashed up the stairs, not knowing where Billy was. On the way up I spotted him, he had found Melissa. They both looked very happy and excited, but I could tell they were trying to stay at arms length. I assumed it was to avoid any problems, that was just the way things were. When Billy spotted me he broke away to join me on stage. We were shouting, "We did it!"

We clowned to the audience and they loved it. The emcee was saying, "Let's hear it for these kids!" The applause was like thunder. It was magnificent.

The all-around championship was yet to be named, but nothing topped the wild Lindy Hop competition that night. The Lindy Hoppers under Whitey would hold that record for fourteen out of the next sixteen years. The Lindy Hop competition belonged to us. That night Whitey's Lindy Hoppers were born. We entered the Garden as the Savoy Lindy Hoppers, but left as Whitey's Lindy Hoppers.

THE SWINGIN' GENERATION

The victory at the Harvest Moon Ball put Whitey on top as far as Lindy Hop dancing was concerned, but rumors were flying, and supposedly they were coming out of the mayor's office. Action was being taken to keep the (white) downtown money from flowing uptown to Harlem. White businessmen had been unhappy about Harlem being New York's playground for quite some time, and the dissatisfaction was increasing.

There was also a lot of concern about situations like Billy and Melissa's—nice white girls coming to dance in Harlem. The interracial dancing could not be stopped because the ballroom was integrated, but closing down the Savoy would eliminate the problem. It was suggested that if they could link the Savoy to prostitution, the shutdown could be accomplished quickly. Moe Gale caught wind of this and called a meeting with Charlie Buchanan.

The story that circulated later went something like this. Charlie Buchanan was in his office, counting the weekend receipts when Moe Gale arrived, looking very serious. As usual, his pipe was jutting from the side of his mouth, but his jaw was set tight and his brow was furrowed.

Mr. Gale asked Charlie to put the receipts away for a minute and come into his office where Moe informed Charlie of the situation. He told him they were hearing rumors about the hostesses. He said he knew where they were coming from, but they were going to have to be very careful. People in power were looking for any reason to close down the Savoy.

Charlie said he was aware of what was being said, but played down the rumors; they had nothing to do with their hostesses. He believed they couldn't stand Negroes having a nice ballroom. He believed they also resented the fact that white folks were coming uptown to the Savoy; they just didn't like seeing the ballroom succeed.

Mr. Gale agreed but reminded Charlie that the authorities would probably do whatever they could to discredit the ballroom. He told Charlie to mind his Ps and Qs and expect them to try anything. Including cheap shots like accusing their dancers and hostesses of whoring.

Charlie already had a meeting scheduled for that evening. He was determined to get the entire situation under control.

Later that day, while waiting for the meeting to begin, Charlie approached the hostesses' corner to speak with his two favorites; Sissy Bowe, a beautiful woman and former hostess who was now in charge of the candy concessions, and Helen Clarke, a dance hall hostess who had been with the Savoy since Charlie first hired dance hostesses and teachers. Both women were the eyes and ears of the management on the floor. He filled them in on the rumors. Neither knew of anything of the kind going on.

It was nearly time for the meeting to begin and they all headed for the office. Charlie called to Whitey, who was in the corner rehearsing us and asked him to join them. Jack Larue, the head of security joined them as well.

He told them that they would all need to work together or the ballroom could be in a lot of trouble. He knew that they had all heard rumors about people wanting to close the Savoy down. He said that anything that might be construed as the girls dating customers would stop immediately. He didn't want to hear about any of the hostesses going with the boys from Yale . . . or anyone else for that matter. He said it was all right to dance with them, that was their job, and they could also give private lessons on Sunday afternoons, they could even take tips, but that was where it ended. Everyone was already aware that dating customers was not allowed. There were to be no second chances, if a hostess dated a customer, she was going to be fired. Immediately. Period. He also didn't want the girls dating the musicians. They were there to play music, the girls were there to entertain customers. He said there were people who'd do anything to close them up, but he wasn't going to give them the chance. So there were the rules. Anyone who couldn't abide by the rules, wouldn't have a job. He said he hoped he was understood.

Everyone agreed and Jack LaRue spoke up letting Mr. B. know he could depend on his guys to do their job. He thought it was a bitch, that the only reason they were after them was to keep white people from coming to Harlem.

The rumor went around that Mr. B had dismissed the meeting, making sure Helen would convey the message very clearly to her girls, then asked Whitey for a moment in private. Charlie said that a lot of people had noticed what was going on between Billy and the young white girl Melissa. Charlie believed that her father was someone of importance, that he might have something to do with the pressure that was being put on the ballroom. Regardless, he wanted Whitey to do what he could to put a stop to it. Right or wrong, they needed to try everything.

Whatever was actually said in that conversation, it was clear that Whitey knew that he had to do something about Billy and Melissa right away. The last thing he needed was a problem over a couple of kids with raging hormones. He also knew that Billy really had a thing for this girl, and it wasn't going to be easy. Whitey decided to deal with Billy when he saw him next.

Anything pertaining to the Lindy Hop, in or out of the ballroom came under Whitey's direction. He decided Shorty Snowden could keep whatever gig he had going, but all future bookings would be his. Leon James may have won the Harvest Moon's first prize, but Whitey held its diamond ring. Now he could build his Lindy Hop dynasty.

Shortly after the ball, the Savoy began to receive calls requesting Lindy Hoppers at clubs and theaters. The Gale Agency also began to package Lindy Hoppers into the band tours it arranged.

One of the first calls Whitey received was for a tour of several European countries, including England, France, and Switzerland. He lined up Leon with his partner Edith, who were both eager to go to Europe.

Whitey asked Frankie, but Frankie said no. He had a steady job as a furrier and was not willing to give it up for dancing. At the Savoy that evening, Whitey and Frankie argued for several hours, then Frankie left for his girlfriend Dot's apartment. Whitey was not one to take no for an answer. He jumped into his car and drove to Dot's place.

Whitey sat waiting for him on the stoop, and when Frankie arrived, Whitey resumed the argument. They continued to argue until dawn. Frankie never did make it up the stairs that night, but neither did Whitey convince him to go to Europe.

Whitey saw the Europe tour as a perfect opportunity to get Billy out of the country, away from Melissa. He decided to ask Billy and me next. However, Tim Gale, Moe Gale's brother and manager of the Gale Agency, told Whitey that I was going to be a problem. I was under age and still in school, and I was also under the protection of a mother who didn't think she wanted her daughter in the Savoy at all. Gale told Whitey he would not be able to get my mother's permission. Still, Whitey decided to try. First he asked Billy, who surprisingly agreed without hesitation. Then he told me. I was thrilled, but told him I would have to find a way to get my mother's consent.

That night, on the way home from the ballroom, all I could do was try to think of a way to swing it with Mama. I thought of all kinds of elaborate schemes to get her consent, none seemed sure to work. As I reached home, I decided to play it by ear. It was late and Mama was already in bed. As I passed her room to get to mine, she called out to me.

"Bun, could you do me a favor?"

This was good news, a chance to get on her good side. I would have done anything she asked at this point.

"Sure Ma, what can I do for you?"

"Would you wash those things I've got soaking in the sink? I'm too tired to bother with them now."

"Okay Ma, but if I wash out your underwear, will you let me go to Europe?"

Not taking me seriously she said, "Yes Bunny, if you wash those things I'll let you go to Europe."

I washed out her clothes and in the morning she was astonished to find that I was serious. I held her to her promise.

That day Whitey came over to talk with my mother. He could talk anyone into anything. He could really pour on the charm, and he turned on all the faucets in that conversation with my mother. He told Mama that I would be chaperoned, and he convinced her that I wouldn't get into any trouble. At long last she agreed to let me go.

We began preparing for the trip. Passports had to be applied for, there were contracts to be signed, and new costumes to be made. I even got a brand new outfit and my first pair of high Cuban heels to wear socially. After all, we were going to dance in a theater for the first time. The contract was for two weeks at the Piccadilly Theater in London, with an option to stay over. I asked Tim Gale, who was to be our chaperon on the trip, what that meant. He told me that if we were successful, our engagement would continue after the two weeks.

Throughout the weeks of preparation I was forbidden to breathe a word to anyone about the trip, even my best girlfriends. It was pure torture, here was the most exciting thing that had happened in my life, and I had to keep my lips sealed.

We never told my school that I was leaving. My mother agreed not to say anything, but she also said that when the truant officer came, she would not lie to him. I agreed to that. I had just started at Textile High in September; Textile was not the best school to attend. It had limited programs and was located on top of an elementary school. I had requested permission to go to a better high school with more liberal programs, but because of zoning, my request was denied. As much as I had always enjoyed school, at that point I lost interest in it. My formal education was ending, but life on the road would teach me a lot.

We sailed on a Friday night in October. I spent my last day in school acting as normally as possible, and saying nothing to anyone. At three o'clock as I was leaving school I looked at all of my class mates for the last time. I quietly picked up my books and walked out. By the time school would begin again on Monday, I would be well past the Statue of Liberty and in the middle of the Atlantic Ocean!

When I arrived home from school the apartment was already full of well wishers. Although the trip had not been mentioned to my own friends, Mama's pals were well aware of it. Our home was always full of Mama's wild friends and this was certainly reason for a party. The cocktails were flowing, and the entire group accompanied me to the docks. There we met Whitey, Frankie, and all the Lindy Hoppers along with other friends and relatives who were there to see us off.

I was taken on a tour to find our cabin, and Mama and several of her friends followed me. When I came back up on deck to join the bon voyage party, it was nearly time to sail, and the crew was asking all visitors to leave the ship. I looked everywhere for Mama to say goodbye until I found out where she was. She had fallen asleep in my cabin!

Several of us went to wake her and get her off the ship before we were charged with a stowaway. I shook Mama a couple of times before she opened her eyes.

"Bunny, you're still here" she said.

"Mama, you're on the ship. You gotta get outta here so we can sail!"

"Oh damn! Why'd you let me fall asleep?" she grumped, scrambling to get up.

We all laughed and hurried back on deck. When we got to the gangplank Dot was still there waiting for Mama. We all hugged and said our goodbyes. The mood was gay, I was thrilled to be going to Europe, and they couldn't help but be happy for me.

That night, everything changed. I was entering an adult world where I was expected to be on my best behavior at all times.

The S.S. *Berengaria,* a Cunard ship, sailed at midnight as scheduled. We didn't really get a chance to see the ship until the next day. The call for breakfast gave us our first chance to see the other passengers and gave them a chance to see us. Being the only black people on board, we really stood out.

We went to the dining room for our meal. The room was lovely, and I was nervous, never having been in a formal dining room before. When my eggs were served I was surprised to see that they were sunny side up. I had never seen eggs like that. They looked like two glossy yellow eyeballs staring up at me from my plate, not appetizing at all. So I decided to eat my roll first. Now, I was used to soft biscuits, that you cut open, but when I put my knife to the roll, it was hard. The pressure sent the roll sailing through the air, landing far from our table. I was sure the whole dining room had seen, and my face burned with embarrassment. Thankfully, the waiter came almost immed-

iately and without a word put a fresh roll on my plate. That
morning I learned to break bread.

It didn't take long before the other passengers knew who
we were. Being a troupe of dancers made us a curiosity, and
every day the ship's crew asked when we would perform for
the other passengers.

Dancing on a ship can be very difficult. Even though it
was a large ship, it was in constant motion. Therefore we
were constantly adjusting our balance—and that wasn't the
worst part. The worst part was the music. Up until then we
had danced mostly at the Savoy, and we knew all the bands,
all the musicians, all the music, all the solos, and all the riffs.
Even at the Harvest Moon Ball, our first dance outside the
Savoy, we danced to Fletcher Henderson's swing band. But
this, this was different. The band, a small, four-piece British
combo, had no concept of swing. The drummer had a
rickety, ticky sound with no push and no beat. We didn't
even know that there was popular music that didn't swing.
It was appalling.

We gave two performances in the dining room, one for
first class and one for economy. Naturally, Leon was wonderful. He won them over, his wiggly legs, his irrepressible
smile, and his pointing finger always dazzled an audience.
He and Edith looked like the champions they were. Billy
and I took our turn, doing our best to swing to the tinny
tune, but there wasn't much of a beat to swing to. The
passengers seemed to be amused, but we thought they were
just being polite. We thought it was awful.

"It ain't the track," we told each other afterwards.

Somehow we got through it, but it was an omen of
things to come. We realized we were at the mercy of

whatever band we were working with. Dancing the Lindy
Hop was a very emotional thing, and a good swinging
drummer could make you sail through a routine, you never
got tired because everything was in synch. But this, this was
a dance trial.

Seven days later we arrived at Dover and then took the
train to London where we were welcomed by theater
people. The Four Flash Devils, a top dance team, invited us
to the Palladium where they were performing with the
comedy team Beatty and Foster, with Gracie Fields as the
star act.

I was very excited and put on my best new outfit and my
high Cuban heels. I was pleased with the way I looked; I
wanted to make an impression on London.

When we entered the Palladium I was impressed. Taking
everything in, I neglected to watch my step and tripped
over my own two feet. I did a belly dive and slid right into
the lobby! I thought I'd die; I wasn't sure whether to laugh
or cry. Billy rushed to my aid, and after making sure I was
okay, he burst out laughing. I joined in and we laughed so
hard I could barely get to my feet. This was my grand
introduction to London night life.

We enjoyed the show that night and returned early to
our rooms. We all needed rest. The next day we went to
the theater, where it was even more intimidating. Unlike
the Savoy, it was cold and huge. There would be no friends
in the audience to inspire us, there was only the four of us
dancers and Tim Gale.

We were backing up a very popular American act, the
Kentucky Singers. They were a well known quartet of
spiritual singers who had performed at the theater before.

They wore white tails on stage, performing in the stiff, square style that had been coming from America to England. It wasn't finger-poppin' stuff, but they had good harmony.

Our act followed theirs, and it was even worse than on shipboard. The band was in the pit. It sounded a hundred miles away, and didn't have an ounce of swing.

Billy and I danced first. Billy bucked his eyes, and I did my best to make the audience laugh, but they just stared. They looked like a landscape, not living, breathing people. When Leon and Edith swung out, the audience gave them a polite reception. When we retired backstage we were completely dejected. Tim Gale saw us all sitting around in a funk and tried to cheer us up. He told us that the British were different, they just didn't give in to their emotions the way Americans did. He said he was sure that they really loved us, they just reacted differently.

Maybe he was right, we didn't know. Regardless, it was no help. We were used to an audience who sat on the floor and egged us on, screaming at the top of their lungs. An audience that did everything but join the dancing.

We managed to survive two weeks of polite applause, mostly because evenings we would escape to Ike Hatch's Nest Club in the West End. Hatch was a black American entertainer who had come over some years before and had opened this club. It was a place for Americans to hang out. We spent time there every night, and we met some of the famous black acts that I had heard about in the halls of Textile High, as well as some royalty. Still, it was a poor substitute for the Savoy.

Ike Hatch also owned the London Shim Sham Club. It

was there that I met Henry Wilcox, the English actor. He was a lot of fun, and we spent many nights hanging out together. One particular night at the Shim Sham Club, I had taken a seat at the bar where drinks were prepared and all lined up, they looked like iced tea. The bartender wasn't there, and I was thirsty, so I grabbed one of the drinks and started gulping. When I stopped to take a breath, I realized I was definitely not drinking iced tea. Whatever it was, it was awful. I nearly gagged. Henry, who had tried to warn me before I took the drink, told me it was scotch and soda. He was laughing so hard he practically fell off his stool. It was not a pleasant introduction to scotch, something I've never acquired a taste for.

Next Gale booked us into a series of ballrooms, scattered throughout the provinces surrounding London. Here we were to demonstrate the dance and then give the patrons a Lindy Hop lesson. The British ballrooms were very formal; the women wore gowns and the men, tuxedos. We entered our first British ballroom in our little costumes to see gowned ladies twirling to a waltz—and nearly got thrown out. When Billy and I performed, we let out our usual yells as we swung out, and it just about scared the hell out of them.

The booking wasn't great, but it was better than the Piccadilly Theater. The band was used to playing for dancers and could swing a bit more. After our exhibitions, we would break up, and each of us would dance with the patrons for the rest of the night. It was very odd to see ladies in gowns swing-out, but they enjoyed it. Thus began the introduction of the Lindy Hop to England.

Our next stop was in Switzerland where we picked up a

"The Horse was a step that we, the Lindy Hoppers, created."

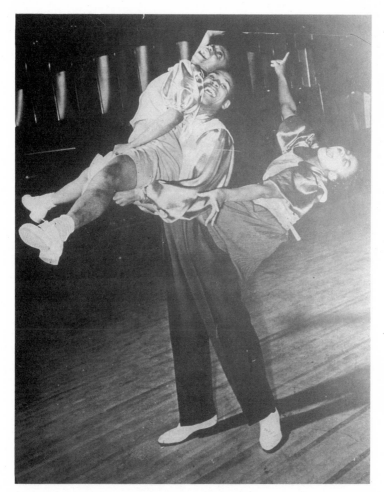

The Horse, as danced by Norma Miller, William Downes, and Joyce James (front to back).

trumpet player named Jack Hammer. He played in the band and was a big asset. He had been stranded in Zurich and spoke several languages. We thought that he would really be of help while we were traveling in Europe. Unfortunately, his passport was being held by the authorities because he had run up some huge debts, and they didn't want him to leave the country without paying them. He and Gale struck some kind of deal, and it was agreed that if he could get to Paris, we'd guarantee him a job with our show. We took his trumpet with us while he snuck across the border.

When we boarded the train everything went smoothly. As we neared the border, the customs inspectors were making rounds, and they stopped to ask if we knew Jack Hammer. We said we did not. While we were being questioned, I noticed that the trumpet in our luggage had Hammer's name clearly printed on it! Fortunately, the customs official didn't notice it, and, when we finally arrived in Paris, we found Hammer waiting for us. He had somehow managed to arrive before we did.

In Paris we performed at the Bal Negre, along with a series of other black acts. I had two numbers as a singer, "Red Sails in the Sunset" and "You are my Lucky Star." Our Paris stay was the best of the whole trip. In our spare time we would frequent the cafés and talk with the locals. There were many young black Frenchmen who spent time in the cafés, and they befriended us. Most of them were very political. They told us stories of prejudice—worldwide prejudice of which we had been completely unaware. One of the main concerns was South Africa and the conditions there. They told us what items and brands were coming out of South Africa, and we joined them in their boycott.

Just being in Paris was an education. Rather than sitting
in a history class in New York, I was getting my lessons first
hand. The Parisians were very friendly, and I took great joy
in slipping away from my group and seeing the landmarks
and museums with a knowledgeable citizen.

At the end of June we sailed for New York. Mother and
Dot were waiting for me when I arrived. Back in October,
they had put a fifteen-year-old Bunny on a boat to dance in
Europe, but when I walked off that ship, I believed I was
the Grand Dame. I had turned sixteen while in Europe, and
I had performed in grand theaters, I had visited clubs in
London, Switzerland, and Paris, and had been in the most
famous museums, I was bigger than life itself. . . . Somehow
I had forgotten just who my Mama was. While we were
waiting for a taxi, I asked for a cigarette; a man standing
nearby was happy to oblige, and Dot made the mistake of
giving me a light. Mama snatched the cigarette from my
mouth and let us both have it, right there on the street,
quickly putting an end to my nonsense.

That evening Whitey took us down to see his other dancers, Frankie and Naomi, Lucille and Jerome, and Billy and
Millie, who were performing at the Apollo. We didn't
know what to expect. We heard the music start and Boom!
the three teams came out. Not only had their routines
changed, but, unbelievably, they were all dancing together!
While we were gone, the Lindy Hop had changed.

When we left for Europe, Whitey began getting the
others jobs around town. Frankie had been able to dance at
night and still keep his job in the fur trade. This worked out
well for everyone. It also got Shorty Snowden's attention.

Shorty had said that he wanted to challenge Whitey's dancers to a contest, to be held, of course, at the Savoy. It would be a big battle, the grand old man of the Lindy Hop against the young upstarts. Each side would have three teams dancing separately.

Frankie chose Frieda Washington as his partner. They were a great team for contests, and it was particularly convenient because they both lived on 140th Street, two doors from each other. They both lived on the top floor, so they could go over the roof to either of their apartments to rehearse.

Frankie, always the innovator, decided to try something new for this contest. Shorty Snowden and his partner, Big Bea, would end their routine with her carrying him off the stage on her back. Frankie decided to improve on this by taking Frieda all the way over his back, making it into a step, and doing it in time with the music. Frieda, being daring, agreed to try it. They had no acrobatic training, so it was difficult at first. They linked arms back to back, Frankie bent over, and Frieda rolled off his back. They would fall and try it over again. Many bruises later, they got it. Frankie then figured out how they could get into and out of it, staying with the music. They called it Over the Back. It was the first aerial step in Lindy.

Frankie and Frieda kept the new step to themselves. They wanted to save it as a surprise for the contest. They didn't even tell Whitey. The Thursday evening of the contest, Leroy and Bea danced first, then Billy and Millie, next Freddie and his sister, and then Jerome and Lucille. Shorty, being the best dancer and the leader of his trio danced last, even though his style was comical, which would normally be seen first. That threw him up against Frankie and Frieda. Shorty and Big Bea went first and did their usual routine, it was great and the crowd burst into applause.

Frankie and Frieda were excited because they knew they had something that no one had done before. They did their routine and then went into the new step. She flew over his back, "Boom!" Then she stood up, fell on him into the jig walk position, and they jigged off the stage. The audience roared.

Whitey ran and embraced them, he was grinning from ear to ear. The young dancers were shouting, "That was great! That was amazing!" jumping up and down around them, demanding to be taught the new step.

The whole Savoy crowd was still screaming, they had forgotten about Shorty Snowden and the others. When Charlie Buchanan finally got their attention, he said, "We'll have to give this contest to the youngsters." Even Shorty Snowden swallowed his pride and congratulated them.

That was just the beginning of the aerial steps. Frankie continued to create more, such as Over the Shoulder. Everyone wanted to learn them. The development of aerial steps was one of two major changes to the Lindy in the Spring of 1936. The other was ensemble dancing. Until then, Lindy Hop couples had danced by themselves, one after another, but never in an ensemble. Once again, Frankie Manning was the genius behind the change. He got the idea one evening while dancing to Jimmy Lunceford's number, "For Dancers Only," during which the music stops; so when it did, Frankie would stop too. He suggested to Whitey they make it an ensemble dance in which everyone would do the same steps. Whitey thought it sounded great, so Frankie took it further by adding these stops to music that didn't stop, to numbers such as "Christopher Columbus." The dance routine became known as the Stops.

Several weeks later, Whitey was contacted by the director of the Cotton Club show that was being performed at the Alhambra who had decided to take on a Lindy Hop act. It was a perfect place to introduce the new version of the dance. When it came time for their act, the dancers started doing their improvisations, one after another, as had been done before. Then, when the last couple performed, they all gathered around and jockeyed until they were all together. Then they all swung out into their prearranged routine, with the stops.

This actually stopped the Cotton Club show! Not an easy feat. The audience continued applauding wildly until the dancers had to go back for an encore. When they were finished, they were so happy with what they'd done that they strutted down 125th Street, high as the breeze. They were all looking in store windows and saying, "Man, I'm gonna buy this, and this, and this. . . ." They were being paid forty dollars each, and they felt they were in the show for good. Considering you could have a suit tailor made for $27.50 at Wilma's, they were on easy street.

The group walked back to the theater, happy and jolly, their heads full of big ideas. As they were preparing to go back on stage, the manager called Frankie over. He assumed it was to compliment them, or even give them a raise. Instead, he told them they were out of the show.

Frankie stared in disbelief. He argued with the manager,

telling him he was crazy, that the audience had loved them. The manager said he didn't have time to discuss it and walked away.

The group was stunned and hurriedly called Whitey at the Savoy. He immediately came over to argue with the director. He was told the group was fired because the show was too long, but the dancers heard that it was because they had stopped the show, and they didn't want anybody from outside the Cotton Club stopping the Cotton Club show.

Under Whitey's pressure, the manager gave the group another date a month later, with Bunny Briggs. After that, Clarence Robinson, who was the Cotton Club choreographer, worked with them and brought them into the downtown show, when the Cotton Club moved to 48th Street. Ensemble dancing helped make the Lindy Hop suitable for the theater. It was one of the most important steps in the evolution of the dance.

Each of Whitey's dancers was unique, and we never copied each other's steps. That was taboo, dancers were known by the steps they created. The fact that you never saw two teams alike made it exciting. The dancers' nicknames were taken from their steps. There was Snookie Beasley's famous "lock step" in which he swung the girl around and reversed, throwing her weight such that he is able to lean on her with his legs twisted like a lock. There was Long George (Greenwich), who, because of his long legs, did his Charleston Split. Of course there was Stompin' Billy, who had a way of slapping his foot that brought the house down. Then there was Leon James with his Wiggly Legs that could never be duplicated. These were the things that made each dancer's Lindy Hop distinct.

Whitey's Lindy Hoppers had a very special place in the
life of the Savoy. We were the favorites of the staff and the
tourists alike. The presence of the dancers was as important
to the ballroom as the music, because without the dancer's
reaction to the music, the Savoy would not have been as
popular as it was. There was a particular interaction between the music and dancing that stood out; it was a
confrontation. Whitey became the Lindy Hopper's benefac-
tor and, for the first time, came to our defense.

A night billed as the greatest battle of the bands was
announced. It was to be a battle between the giants of
swing, Count Basie and Chick Webb. Both bands were
popular, but Chick was the boss in the ballroom. To get
your "Swing wings" you had to take on a giant like this
cocky, five foot bundle of dynamite. A master at drums,
Chick Webb was the best and the quickest, and if anyone
disagreed with that, Mr. Webb would tell them in a minute
what to do with their opinion.

One afternoon in the ballroom we were all milling about,
discussing the upcoming events. Nothing could get a bunch
of Lindy Hoppers off and running like a question about
music, and who swings better than whom. This time the
talk was about a new sound coming from Kansas City from
the Count Basie Band.

The dancers were around Cissy's counter and the first
booth, talking about the battle that was going to take place.
We were like a gang, a dancing gang. We discussed bands as
if they were our own personal property. Some dancers liked
the sounds of Chick Webb, some liked Duke Ellington,
whatever the preference, it always ended up in an argument.

Snookie brought a record in and was telling us about the

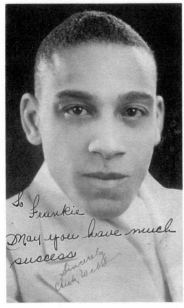

"chick was the bandleader who introduced ella fitzgerald. After his death, she led the band for some time. This photo is from frankie manning's collection."

Chick Webb, whose band was often the house band at the Savoy.

"Thelma was the first black to play on prime-time radio; she was with the eddie canton show. she used to play vegas in the old days."

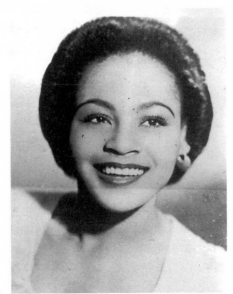

Thelma Carpenter.

new sound. He was saying we'd better listen to this cat, that he could really swing. Snookie had a funny way of speaking as much with his hand gestures as his words. I looked at him, wondering if he would be able to speak without his hands, when someone asked what the band was like and brought my attention back to the music.

Snookie said that to him, Basie had a real bluesy sound, but it swung. Snookie was always the one to bring us up to date on anything, especially the bands. And he was usually right. He told us that the little guy—meaning Webb—was going to be in trouble.

That was often said about Chick Webb, but he had his defenders in the group. Someone always stood up and said that Chick didn't have to worry about anybody, that he was the swingingest in the joint. But Snookie insisted that there was a new sound coming, and Mr. Basie was going to upset everything when he got there.

This conversation was somehow blown all out of proportion when it got back to Chick Webb himself. When he heard it, it sounded like the kids were saying he didn't have it anymore, and that the sound the Basie band was bringing would run him off the bandstand. Now, Chick Webb was usually the one to do the running off, usually running the bands right back to where they came from.

Of course, when Chick heard of this he responded in typical Chick Webb fashion saying, "I don't give a good God damn what those raggedy Lindy Hoppers think or say. Who needs them? As far as I'm concerned they can all go to hell, and that goes for their mammies too!"

When he turned around, he saw Whitey standing there. They looked each other in the eye, neither saying anything.

Chick looked at Whitey as if to say, "Well, I said it, take it or leave it." Then he shrugged and walked off with that strange pulled-up pants look of his.

Whitey watched him walk away. He was steaming, but he kept his cool. Nothing was said, and everything seemed to get back to normal. The incident was forgotten until the night of the big bash. Everybody was talking about the bands. There was always excitement when a new band came to town, and this time the band was Count Basie's. There was a coolness between the Lindy Hoppers and Chick Webb, and everybody thought it was the excitement of the evening.

The surprise came later that night. As we entered the ballroom, Whitey met us and he told us that when Chick got on the bandstand, all dancers were to leave the floor.

Talk about a shock! The corner was utterly quiet, and that was strange, but as the night began, no one noticed anything. The Basie band hit the stand, and everything was jumping, the floor was crowded with dancers. As soon as Chick Webb went up, the corner went still. No dancers at all. Chick tried to act as though nothing was amiss, but as the evening wore on, it became obvious to everyone, including Charles Buchanan—Whitey was showing Chick that he did need the dancers.

Here were the two favorites in the ballroom, going at each other. Buchanan brought the warring parties together and made them both realize that they were important to each other. Whitey had Chick's back against the wall, and Chick was fighting mad, but Chick had to concede to Whitey and was forced to apologize to both Whitey and the Lindy Hoppers. Whitey had proven his point. He had flexed his muscles and won. His dancers were going to be famous and he was going to get the everyone's respect.

After that, Whitey lifted his prohibition on dancing for Webb's band, and we took to the floor when he hit the bandstand. After all, the Lindy Hoppers and Chick's band were a great team, but that night proved that the Basie band would be a favorite of the Lindy Hoppers.

Chick Webb and the Lindy Hoppers soon made up and began performing together again. Years later the Lindy Hoppers performed at his last concert. We also auditioned at the Paramount Theater to work in his show with Ella Fitzgerald. We had become her favorite act because we would play cards with her backstage. She loved the game of Hearts called Dirty Hearts, and she would have a game going after every show.

Our appearing at the Paramount depended on our being able to work on an extension of the Paramount stage that was raised by a hydraulic lift after the picture was over. The difficulty was to not hit Chick's drums, which sat right down front. We pulled off the audition and got the job. It was Chick's final engagement. He became ill during a performance and was taken off stage after the second show. However, there is truth in the old adage that the show must go on, and Kaiser Marshall replaced him in the third show and finished out the engagement.

Shortly after, Chick died of tuberculosis of the spine. Ella was elevated to the titular head of the band, and it became "Ella Fitzgerald and the Chick Webb Band, lead by Bardu Ali." Chick Webb was a great performer, and he was sadly missed by all.

THE OTHER SIDE OF THE BALLROOM

Stretching an entire city block from 140th Street to 141st Street on Lenox Avenue, the Savoy Ballroom had two very distinct sides. The 141st Street side was called "the corner," and it belonged to the professional Lindy dancers. It was, in its way, sacred. Here Whitey's group worked out their intricate routines. This was Whitey's territory, and you had to be a Whitey's Lindy Hopper to dance there. Dancing at the Savoy became a spectator sport. We were the crowd pleasers, and the tourists who came by the bus load, would thrill to our antics.

Press agents saw the value of having stars come to the ballroom. The boxes were reserved for them, and stars such as Alice Faye, Lana Turner, Greta Garbo, Marlene Dietrich, and Delores Del Rio, the latter on the arm of Orson Wells, came to the Savoy. Everybody and his brother came, and they all converged on the 141st Street side to watch the dancers. There was no doubt about it, the crazy Lindy Hoppers were a main attraction at the ballroom.

However, that was just one side of the ballroom. At the other end, on the 140th Street side, a quieter dance was going on. Couples who wanted a bit of privacy liked this side of the ballroom. This was where you would find The Sheik, who used this corner for his ballroom dancing. You could see him gliding across the floor, sometimes twirling his girl in the air. His Tango was always a beautiful sight to see.

The diversity of the dancers made the ballroom swing nightly. The professional hostesses were there for the guys who came without partners and were paid twenty-five cents for each dance. To work as a hostess at the Savoy one had to be well groomed, beautiful, intelligent, and a good dancer. She had to be versatile, not only capable of doing the latest dances, but proficient in the other dances as well; the Waltz, Tango, Rhumba, and Shag. She also had to be able to teach those dances. If she was good at her work, she was awarded at the end of the night with a very good tip.

Dating a customer or fraternizing with the musicians was unacceptable and could result in dismissal. Mr. B seemed to have eyes in the back of his head, and he made sure that no one broke his rules. He made certain there were never any scandals attached to the people who worked at the Savoy. He was considered a slave driver, but he got good results. You were usually so busy working when in the ballroom, that you didn't have time to court trouble. In all the years Mr. B ran the ballroom, it was considered the best run establishment in the city.

Of course, regardless of the rules, a little consorting between hostesses and musicians was inevitable. The key was not getting caught. Often, hostesses would go to the Britwood after work. It was a club on the corner of 140th Street, downstairs from the Savoy, and it was a favorite of the musicians as well. The club was open until four A.M., and they served liquor, whereas the Savoy only served beer and wine. Of course, it was unthinkable for a hostess to drink even these while working. So the Britwood was a place to unwind and mingle after work.

Helen Clarke had been a dance hall hostess since 1931. She supervised the hostesses and worked closely with Charles Buchanan. During her years at the Savoy, she had danced with some very interesting men including Winthrop Rockefeller, Hoagie Carmichael, the young Ezra Stone, and the very dashing Ricardo Cortez, a marvelous dancer. Many kinds of women worked as hostesses at the Savoy. The money was good, and some were taking care of their families. Many hostesses dreamed of meeting and marrying a wealthy or famous patron, and others were just having a good time. The stories are countless.

The fellas from Yale would come down every weekend and go Shag crazy. They were a favorite group. Hostesses from the Roseland Ballroom would also frequent the Savoy. The Roseland, which had a strictly white clientele, did not welcome the Savoy hostesses as guests in their ballroom. So, instead, the Roseland hostesses would come to the Savoy on Monday nights, their night off. This led to Mr. B's Monday-Ladies-Free Nights. There was already a Thursday night ritual called Kitchen Mechanics Night which was for the women who rattled those pots and pans, the domestics. Thursday nights were already very popular, and Mondays were an instant success. The girls came in droves, and naturally the guys—who paid full fare—followed.[1]

Mondays and Thursdays, the Savoy was the place to be. Tuesday nights the Savoy became the watering hole for the 400 Club, a group of regulars who had formed a social club.

1. Clarke interview.

They all wore yellow and green corduroy jackets with "400 Club" on the back, and they held informal dance contests. Tuesday nights became so popular that Willie Bryant even broadcast a live radio show from the Savoy those evenings called *The 400 Club*. Wednesday and Friday nights Mr. B reserved for gala community affairs. When the savoy first opened, Buchanan's idea was to make it a community center as well as a ballroom. Harlem social clubs and fraternal groups held meetings there. The first Miss Colored America Beauty Pageant held its finals at the Savoy. The Urban League gave their Beaux Arts Ball there yearly. The Savoy sponsored numerous benefits and charity dances. It was also known for special promotions; at one time, an automobile was given away every Saturday night to a lucky ticket holder. At Thanksgiving and Christmas the Savoy gave dinners away to needy families.

There was also the political aspect of the Savoy. Far removed from the regular scene, various political groups held meetings there. Charlie Buchanan was heavily involved in this facet of ballroom activities. He was actually a fascinating man—an ex-socialist organizer and later publisher of the *People's Voice* in association with Adam Clayton Powell. It was the most progressive newspaper in Harlem.

The great jazz impresario John Hammond also had a column in the *People's Voice* in which he attempted to tell the truth about the terrible exploitation of black artists, not only in Harlem but everywhere. Hammond, a white man and a Yale graduate, was a regular at the Savoy. He became a close friend of Charlie Buchanan, Moe Gale, and Joe Geleski—Gale's uncle and silent partner in the Savoy. John Hammond formed the Benny Goodman band in 1933

"There was nothing small about their sound."

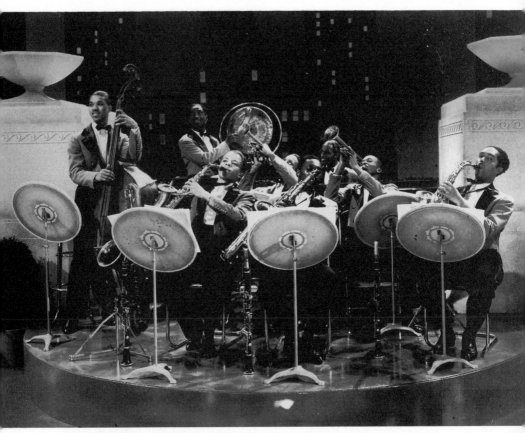

The original Savoy Sultans, who were the house band for the Savoy's small
bandstand during the 1940s.

when he was just twenty-two. He knew that the black and
white musicians had to come together if the music was to
progress, and he began fighting for more integration. From
the beginning, John wanted the Benny Goodman band to
be integrated, but Goodman was scared because New York
was as Jim-crowed as Alabama in its own way. Hammond
was the man responsible for booking the Goodman band for
the great battle against Chick Webb in 1938. He was the
first to bring musicians like Fletcher Henderson, Lionel
Hampton, Teddy Wilson, and Charlie Charitain to the
listening public and the first to recognize the talents of,
among others, Billie Holiday, Lester Young, and Aretha
Franklin. He got Billie Holiday her first recording contract.

Hammond saw the future of good music dependant upon
free racial interaction, he knew change was needed if this
music was to survive. Music was segregated only by habit.
Black musicians played with black bands. White musicians
played society swing. Hammond knew that there had to be

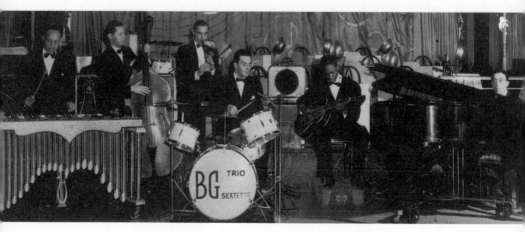

The Benny Goodman Sextet.

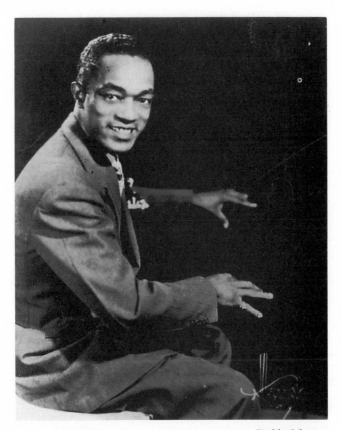

Buddy Johnson.

"He will go out playing drums; lots of people associate him with vibes, but his first love was drums."

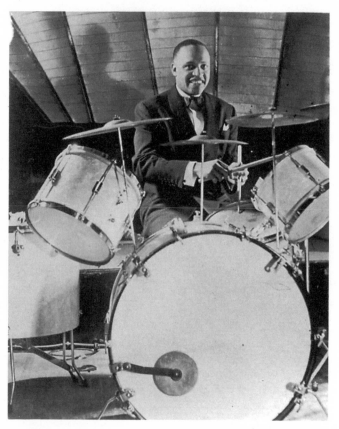

Lionel Hampton.

"JUNE WAS A big WOMAN, AND she made a joyful sound."

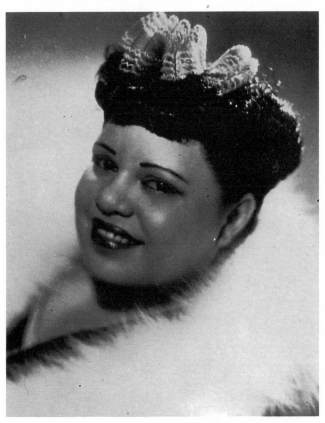

June Richmond, who sang with Andy Kirk and his Clouds of Joy.

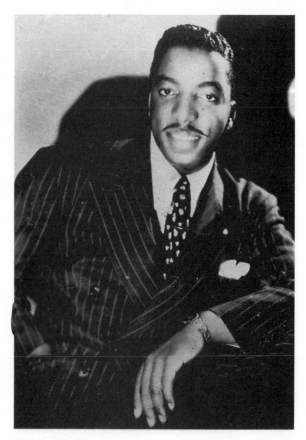

Erskine Hawkins.

"He was known as 'the twentieth-century Gabriel'."

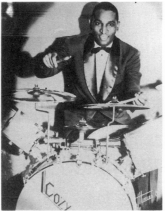

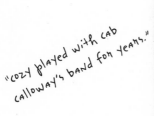

"Cozy played with Cab Calloway's band for years."

Cozy Coles.

a blending of the music as well as of the races. He knew his job was monumental, but no one was better equipped with the tenacity and fortitude the job required than Hammond. He saw what had to be done and did it. He was one of the many important people in jazz who had a lifetime pass to the Savoy. As he said, "Swing may not have been invented at the Savoy, but it matured there."[2]

Harlem was the birthplace of Swing and the Savoy was its incubator. At any given time at the Savoy you could see something or someone of importance. The big bands came and brought their own audience. It was an important step for a band to play the Savoy, because the Savoy bestowed upon them the medal of Swing. It carried a band everywhere else. The big white bands came to the ballroom as well as the bands traveling through. The music inspired the dancers, and the dancers inspired the music.

2. John Hammond, jazz impresario, personal interview, 1982.

117

Bob Bailey was born in Detroit in 1927 and raised in Cleveland. He attended college in Atlanta, which, strangely, led to his singing for the Count Basie Band. A show playing the Moulin Rouge took him to Las Vegas in 1955, and he decided to make Vegas his home. Bob still did some traveling, managing Pearl Bailey on the road for three years. After hosting his own television show and doing some work in radio, Bob returned to business school. After many successful entrepreneurial ventures, he became head of the Nevada Economic Development Corporation (NEDCO), a company that arranged government funding for minority businesses. From there he went to Washington where he was appointed deputy director of the Minority Business Development Administration (MBDA) by President Bush. Mr. Bailey is still involved in Washington, spending a week out of every month working there. His home base is still Las Vegas where he lives with his wife, Ann.

> *I was singing at a local nightclub in Atlanta on weekends when I was discovered by Benny Goodman and John Hammond who were on a quest for new voices. They were trying to find a pop singer who would fit with the Basie band. They had Jimmy Rushing, who was the star singer with the band, but they needed a ballad singer for the new audiences that Basie would be playing to at the posh hotels he was about to appear in. Basie was going into the Waldorf Astoria Hotel, and the added style was necessary.*
>
> *I had heard of Benny Goodman, but I didn't have a clue who John Hammond was. So, after my first set they invited me over to their table. We made small talk, then John Hammond told me why they were there. He asked if I would like to sing with the Basie band. I was flabbergasted. At the time I was still going to school and would be graduating in June. John suggested I find out*

how many credits I had, maybe I would have enough to graduate in January, or I could join the band and finish my education after a stint with Basie. Of course I would have to go to New York to audition for Basie, they would pay my expenses, and then I could come back to Atlanta and finish out the term.

It was the Christmas holidays, and I was going home to Cleveland to see my folks. On the way back to Atlanta I would stop off in New York to meet with Basie and sing for him, then I would fly back to Atlanta. Well, so much was happening. I had never been on a plane before, I had never been to New York before, never met the great Count Basie before, so my head was spinning like a top.

My interview with Basie was at the R.C.A. Building, atop Radio City. In walked Basie, man oh man. Here I was, a college kid out of Atlanta, meeting with Count Basie and John Hammond. Basie sat at the piano and played for me. Anyone who comes to New York for the first time and not only visits Radio City, but gets to sing there, well, you can never go home again. Nothing was the same after the interview.

When I got back to Atlanta I met with Benjamin Mays, the president of the college. He was terribly disappointed in my leaving to pursue a singing career. It's the old saying, almost, "How you gonna keep 'em down on the farm after they've seen New York?"

I joined the Basie band thinking I would stay for a couple of years and then pick up my scholarship again. Of course, I never went back, my education took a different turn.

Singing with the Basie band took me to the Savoy. This was another mind-blower. The first time I went to the Savoy it was a visit. Buddy Tate took me over. I had never been to Harlem, and I felt the only way to go there was with someone who knew the place. We went up to Harlem, then went straight to the Savoy. I had never seen a ballroom that big in my life. Buddy Johnson was playing there at the time, and Arthur Pryscock was singing. I wanted to see how Arthur handled it. That was when Buddy told me we would be playing there in the next few months. I stood there shocked.

This ballroom was awesome. It just flabbergasted me. The decor, the two bandstands, and the sharpest people I had ever seen before. Plus, all races together. Being from a segregated neighborhood in Cleveland, seeing this just floored me. The ladies were in fabulous gowns, and every man had his shoes shined.

Standing there in front of the bandstand watching Arthur Pryscock and the Buddy Johnson band was one thing. But when I finally got my chance to sing on that bandstand, looking out at all those faces was something else. I didn't believe it. It was one of the greatest moments in my life. A little country boy out of Cleveland, singing at the world famous Savoy Ballroom with the Count Basie Band. It was definitely a mind blowing experience.

—Bob Bailey

ETHEL WATERS

One day when I came into the ballroom, I saw Whitey with the most handsome black woman I had ever seen. She was tall and statuesque with burnt brown skin. I knew immediately I was in the presence of a star. And she was indeed a star, the most famous black woman in the world—Miss Ethel Waters.

Whitey was beaming. You knew when he had that look on his face that a woman had really turned him on. They were speaking softly, I couldn't hear anything they were saying, but Whitey was agreeing to whatever it was.

We were all sitting around, enthralled by her presence. She was exquisite. When Whitey finally called us over to introduce her the guys scrambled to get in front of us. I could easily imagine their thoughts—young, vibrant men looking at a woman of such magnitude. They would be fantasizing about this moment for a long time.

Miss Waters just looked at us with those straight forward eyes of hers. After we were introduced, Whitey had us give her a personal demonstration. Boy, did we swing. After we danced for her, she thanked us, and Whitey escorted her to the door. When he walked back his expression was that of a man completely captivated, hog-tied, and branded.

Miss Waters had visited because the Lindy Hop was popular and she wanted to learn it. She was also thinking of

adding the Lindy Hop to her show. She had come to the
right place and had met the right man. It was agreed that
Miss Waters would come to the ballroom in the evening
and dance with Frankie. Dancing would also be good for
her weight, with which she constantly struggled. She came
to the ballroom that night with her usual escort, Archie
Savage. Frankie danced with her, and I danced with Archie.
Archie and I were friends so it was no hardship, besides
Archie was a good dancer. It was considered best that Miss
Waters go through her paces with Frankie, since Frankie
was the expert and could maneuver her weight. It was
strictly floor dancing, she wasn't going for any prize. She
was the prize and she was to be handled with kid gloves.
For that reason, only Frankie was allowed to dance with her.

We began teaching Miss Waters the Lindy. Usually she
would come in on Friday nights, which were club nights
and less crowded. She didn't dance in the corner, she was
allowed as much room on the floor as she wanted. She was
always a bit of a distraction for the other patrons, but after a
few weeks everyone got used to her being there.

The preparations to add us to her show began, and our
teams were formed. Willamae and Snookie, Ella and Long
George, and Leon and I were partners; we were Whitey's
Lindy Hoppers.

The show that we were to tour with consisted of Derby
Wilson, The Brown Sisters, Eddie Mallory's Band, and a
comedy team. Our first date was at the Apollo with Pigmeat
as the comedy act; from there we played the Howard in
Washington D.C., the Royal in Baltimore, and then we
started on the Paramount circuit. We performed in Cleveland, Columbus, Chicago, and even Los Angeles.

When we arrived in Chicago, Whitey was there to meet us. He would follow us to the different cities in his car. He wouldn't let us go on our own.

He still wanted us to rehearse everyday, but with our schedule it was not an easy thing to do. It was Whitey's way of keeping the reigns pulled tight. He wanted everyone to know that we were still his act. Especially Ethel Waters. Because we had moved into a featured spot in a major show, Whitey had to be sure we wouldn't get any ideas that we could function without him.

In Chicago, our first show was scheduled for ten o'clock in the morning. Whitey made us get up early and rehearse before the early show, complaining that we were getting lazy and that we weren't doing our jobs. After rehearsal he made us walk to work, from the south side of Chicago all the way to the Loop, to the State Theater where we were performing. It was a windy Chicago day, and the air was bitterly cold. It was blowing so hard it nearly lifted me off the street. As we walked, Whitey followed us in the car. We were struggling against the icy wind, which tore at my face. I dared not touch my frozen ears for fear they would shatter.

This walk was supposed to get our blood stirring, but anyone who thought a long, excruciating walk like that could improve our performance had to be out of his mind. I could have killed Whitey. It was the beginning of a growing resentment the dancers felt toward him. We began to resent his being there. It was subtle at first, but we all started to feel like, "Who needs him?" and I think he felt it too.

When we checked into the theater that morning, we looked like we had traveled from the North Pole. Ethel

Waters saw us, and it was obvious that she was mad as hell. She understood the hold that Whitey had over us, and being a compassionate woman, she resented the way he had treated us. She wanted to protect us, but she was smart enough to know not to interfere with Whitey's act. She chose not to say anything then, but wait for a better time.

She began watching us like a hawk. After shows she would call Willamae to her dressing room—she treated her like a daughter. Willamae actually looked like Miss Waters, with her stately carriage and her facial expressions, the resemblance was amazing. We were never included in the visits, but Willamae would come back to our dressing room and tell us what Miss Waters had said. She would ask Willamae questions about our working conditions and was not pleased with what she heard. She felt Whitey was being unfair. Miss Waters and Whitey were two old veterans, and it was inevitable that the two would lock horns over us. We were her star act, and she didn't want anyone, including Whitey, mistreating us.

During an engagement in Cleveland, Miss Waters called the Phyllis Wheately house where we were staying and left instructions for us to meet her at a big department store downtown. We were very surprised and wondered why. When we arrived at the store, we were told to meet her in the coat department where she had us all try on coats. We picked out green coats in all different styles, and she bought one for each of us. All the salespeople in the store were watching. There we were, in the biggest department store in Cleveland with the star, Miss Ethel Waters. The whole store was excited with the event. How lucky could a group of kids be?

This did not sit well with Whitey. He believed that she was trying to take us away from him, that she was trying to buy our love. His was an obsessive jealousy, and this was the first time anyone else had taken care of us. He felt that his authority had been challenged, and it was the beginning of a fight between the two strong personalities.

As kind and compassionate as Miss Waters could be, she had a very short fuse. Many times, as soon as the curtain came down she would turn around and start screaming at full decibel level, "What the fuck was that? Where in the hell did that come from? . . ." She would rant and rave, and often we didn't even know what she was yelling about. We learned not to get in her way. Unfortunately, some of us were slower learners than others.

Miss Waters always had a man traveling with her, but it was difficult for her to find a man of equal status, so she usually supported the men in her life. She seemed painfully aware of this, but Miss Waters always had a firm grip on everything around her, especially her men. During this trip she was with Eddie Mallory, the band leader. One evening as we were preparing to go on stage, the lot of us were in our dressing room when we heard shouting from down the hall.

"If she'll play with those, she'll play with his balls!"

"God help us," I said, "Miss Waters is having a fit."

Just then Ella burst into the room crying and tried to explain what was going on. When she caught her breath she said, "All I did was pick up the weights, I didn't hurt nothin'."

When I asked her what she'd done, she told me she had been walking down the hall when she noticed Mr.

Mallory's dressing room was wide open. There were a bunch of dumbbells lying around, and he had a very large mirror in there. So, she decided to take a look and see what she could lift.

"What in the hell were you thinkin' going into his dressing room?" I asked her. "You don't have any business in there, Miss Waters might just decide to fire you. Damn, if you got her mad enough she might just fire the whole bunch of us!"

She apologized profusely, and, fortunately, Miss Waters dropped it at that. But there were many more tantrums to come.

A battle between Whitey and Miss Waters, these two tyrants, was bound to happen before our closing at the State in Chicago. One morning, when George ordered corn flakes for breakfast, we arrived at the theater to find Miss Waters in a stew about something. Whenever she was bothered by something, everyone walked around on egg-shells. Nobody liked to get Miss Waters' dander up, and it was certainly up this morning.

When the opening was over and we were leaving the wings, we heard Miss Waters say, "And tell Mr. White I want to see him when he gets to the theater!"

We all looked at each other, "Boy something is up."

I said, "Don't ask me, don't start me lying."

It was an expression we used when a question was asked for which we didn't have the answer.

When Whitey arrived at the theater he headed for her dressing room. We were all peeping out of our door. Whitey took off his hat and entered her dressing room, "Yes Miss Waters . . ." and the door closed.

Miss Waters let Whitey have it. Whitey was a scrapper from the old days, and with Miss Waters he was up against a street fighter like himself. This was her show, she paid good salaries to all her cast. She paid Whitey a good salary to supply the Lindy Hoppers for her show. She let him know she didn't like hearing that the dancers weren't making enough money to buy a substantial breakfast.

We heard her say, "You can't do a good show on corn flakes!"

Now we understood what happened and that it was about Long George. The funny thing was, he was just cheap. He could have afforded a better breakfast if he had wanted to have one, but Miss Waters was under a different impression. It lead her to ask just how much Whitey was paying us, and so the two of them had a real blow out.

Nothing was the same after that. We already knew Whitey was being paid more for us than he was giving us. Miss Waters told Willamae how much she was paying Whitey for us, and Willamae knew what we were getting. There was a big difference. This added to the strain between Whitey and his top dance act.

Whitey knew things were coming apart with his top team and began plotting to get other dancers. Of course, we didn't know it at the time, but he wanted to be sure we weren't his only act. He had already been preparing Frankie's group to take over our position. At the time, we were just kids dancing. We knew we had a good act, and we were working with a big star, so we felt we were in show business.

We completed our engagement in Chicago and headed for the Paramount Theater in Los Angeles. It was our first trip to the West Coast, and we were all very excited about going to L.A. We rode on the bus with the rest of the cast, followed by Miss Water's two chauffeured cars, a Lincoln Zephyr and a Lincoln. Whitey followed us in his Buick, and Miss Waters traveled by train.

Traveling on the road was always an experience, but traveling cross-country as a group of black entertainers in 1937 . . . we never knew what we would run into. One particular incident occurred at a White Castle burger stand. We pulled in, a bus load of dancers and musicians, with two chauffeured Lincolns behind us, and were told "We don't serve Negroes here."

One of the musicians came back with, "Well, we don't eat Negroes! Just serve us a burger!"

The restaurant did not give in, and we were turned away. This wasn't unusual. Some places had designated "Negro entrances," but often when we would pull into a town for a break and a bite to eat, we would be directed to a place that would serve us.

Regardless, we were all glad to be journeying out of winter and into sunny California, and we weren't disappointed. When we arrived, we were taken to the Torrence Hotel at 54th Street and Central. There we met Mrs. Torrence, who everyone called Mrs. T., and her beautiful daughter, Lena. California was segregated, and the black area was Central Avenue, California's answer to Harlem.

Our engagement at the Paramount was our last with Miss Waters. Our performance in the show led to our doing the Marx Brothers' movie *Day at the Races*. Whitey had been looking for a chance to get us away from Miss Waters, and the picture deal was it. Now he really had us to himself.

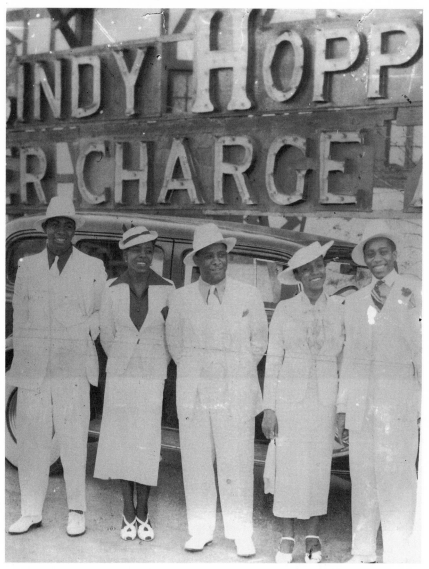

*Whitey, in the middle, and Lindy Hoppers: Snookie Beasley, Willamae
Ricker, Norma Miller, and Leon James, on Easter Sunday, 1937,
in Los Angeles where they were filming* A Day at the Races
with the Marx Brothers.

While we were in California he made sure that we didn't get involved with anyone else. He kept us rehearsing every morning, then we would go to the set and work all day. At night we would go to the Club Alabam where we also performed. It was an exhausting schedule, and we were not being paid for two jobs as normally would be the case. Whitey combined the two and paid us only one salary. We were not stupid, we knew we were worth more, but endured because we had no choice.

The strain between us was obvious. He tried to give us a line about expenses; rent for eight people, transportation. Our pay didn't get any better, but we made it clear to Whitey he couldn't give us a snow job anymore.

The pressure of the schedule and the differences with Whitey had me completely run down. By the time our engagement in California was over, so was my health. I had been unable to eat from the stress, and by the last couple of shows I could barely walk, though somehow I managed to dance. When we returned to New York in July of 1937, I weighed only eighty-seven pounds. I was seventeen years old and completely burned out. My mother immediately put me in the hospital where I was fed intravenously and very slowly nursed back to health.

All of my friends were very supportive. They visited me often in the hospital and kept me up to date. As much as this lifted my spirits, it was five months before I had regained enough physical strength to be released from the hospital. Christmas Day 1937 I was allowed to go home. Mama and Dot came to pick me up, and when I arrived home several of my friends were at our apartment for a small celebration. I was very happy to be home and recovering, but it would take several more months of Mama's cooking before I would be well enough to dance.

In March of 1938 I started dancing again. I was thrilled to be back at the Savoy, and it wasn't long before we had some new excitement. John Hammond was bringing the Goodman band into Harlem to challenge Chick Webb, the undisputed King of Swing, to prove that a white band could swing as well as a black band. He knew that Harlem was the pulse of Swing, and there in the ballroom, all people of all races came together to see good dance and hear good music.

I remember coming into the ballroom and seeing the group of dancers gathered around Cissy's stand. They were talking about the coming event. As usual, Snookie was filling us in on the latest band news. Nothing started us debating like talking about Swing bands. We felt we were the authorities on jazz. It was said that the white boy Goodman had drumming for him was going to put a fire under Chickie boy. Those were fighting words in the ballroom, but no one dared to bet on the outcome.

The big night arrived. The Benny Goodman Band and the Chick Webb Band were both at the peak of their popularity. They were the hottest things in Swing. It was an important night for Goodman, the Savoy, and music. Everyone came to see the battle, an estimated twenty-five thousand packed the place wall to wall. When the bands kicked off, they kicked off with their best Swing tunes, and it stayed like that all night. We danced as if we were in a trance. We never stopped. Both bands pulled out all the stops, and the evening kept on keeping on; the place was swinging! At last Goodman played what the audience had been waiting for all night, "Sing, Sing, Sing." Gene Krupa was warmed up now, and he was sensational. But there was the great Chick Webb, and like he said, "The kid's good, but he's learning, and tonight he'll get his next lesson." Chick Webb let go at the Goodman band with both barrels. The sets kept getting better and better. There was no doubt about it, both bands came away from the ballroom that night with a lot of respect for each other. The night was filled with winners. The people won and the ballroom won. After that, Harlem loved Benny Goodman, because he was a "good man."

My next road trip came when Whitey gave me my own trio and sent us to Canada. I had Downes and Mickey, Joe Daniels and Joyce, and Long George. The resort at which we were performing was in Toronto. Our accommodations were right on the water and it was like heaven. I was elated to be dancing.

SAVOY AT THE WORLD'S FAIR

The coming of the 1939 World's Fair to Flushing, Long Island was hailed as the greatest tribute to mankind and the future. It would unveil the most advanced technology, and it would introduce the newest electronic wonder—television.

Apart from all that the fair would also introduce the world to the dance of the day, the Lindy Hop. The Savoy was going to have its own pavilion where this entirely American dance would be seen nightly. The roots of jazz would also be explained in the Swing show's documentary style. The Lindy Hoppers would be the stars. The ballroom was alive with excitement. To think that the Savoy was to have a ballroom at the World's Fair, it was too fantastic to believe! The fair was to run for six months, and that was the best news of all. We would have steady work and only have to go over the Triborough Bridge to get there, for six months!

The Savoy at the fair would employ two sets of dancers —over forty people. We would have our own ballroom and be given beautiful sets and two bands, Fess Williams and Teddy Hill. Even the musicians were delighted. They too would be working for six months and only have to pay carfare to get to work. Everything was rosy.

Whitey managed the whole production. He and Buchanan were partners in the deal. They had put together the concept. Whitey's star could not have been higher.

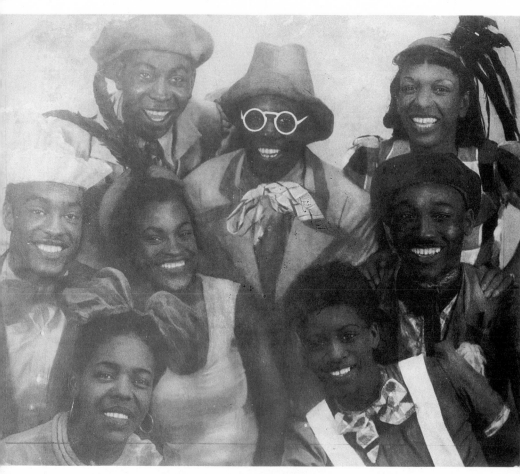

Hollywood Hotel Revue, Billy Ricker, Willamae Ricker, Snookie Beasley, Eunice Callin, Jerome, Lucille Middleton, Frankie Manning, and Esther Washington (left to right).

On an icy day in December we were taken over to
Flushing to the site on which the new Savoy was to be
built. We were there for the ground breaking ceremonies.

There was no music, just a cold ceremony with the usual
speeches. We were all in winter gear, bundled up to the
nostrils, but Whitey made us dance to celebrate the ground
breaking. We lined up with four couples—Mickey and
Downes, Joyce and Joe, Leon and Ann, and George and
me. (Frankie was not there, he was in Australia with the
Hollywood Hotel Revue). We would be opening the fair.
We did our ensemble routine with no specialties. Then the
diggers came in with their shovels. Mr. Buchanan and Moe
Gale dug up the ground, everyone applauded, and then,
thank God, we rushed to the waiting cars. We didn't know
it was an omen.

Whitey was really up there. He had a group in Australia,
another preparing for the greatest fair on earth, and he had
male dancers in *Knickerbocker Holiday*, the Broadway show
starring Walter Houston. Then he got the call from Mike
Todd about the new Broadway show *Hot Mikado*, starring
Bill Robinson.

While Whitey was concentrating on his show at the
World's Fair, he started rehearsing a group for *Hot Mikado*.
Originally it was to have six dance teams, but Whitey
insisted they use seven. The teams were made up of some
leftover dancers, and some new kids who had started
dancing at the Savoy. His main dancers were already
booked, with Frankie Manning's group "down under" and
the rest of us at the World's Fair. Eight of the guys were
tied up in *Knickerbocker Holiday*. At this time Whitey had
dancers all over the country. He had conquered Europe,

Australia, America. He had two movies under his belt, and now he was tackling Broadway. There was no question, he was the dance master of Harlem. Nowhere could you see a swinging black show without the Lindy Hop, whether at the Cotton Club, the Roxy Theater, Radio City, in the *Ethel Waters Show*, the *Hot Mikado*, or Billy Rose's *Casa Manana*.

When the Lindy Hoppers arrived at the first rehearsals for the *Hot Mikado*, the other cast members looked down on them as raggedy dancers from a ballroom. Lindy Hop was not considered show business, and most of the dancers were very young. It was their first time on Broadway, and, at first, they were ostracized. It was overwhelming to them, and Whitey was not there each day to supervise, since he was with his major project, the World's Fair.

We began rehearsing for the fair at the ballroom. It was to be an anthology of the dance, from the roots of black dancing in Africa to the Lindy Hop. The production had an African jungle scene, feathers and all. Tanya danced the African number; she was supposedly a real princess. Whitey was producer, director, and choreographer; in short, the master planner. The overall idea was a good one, because after all, who knew the Lindy Hop better than Whitey? Unfortunately, it was here that his knowledge of choreography and dance stopped, but who would dare tell him?

The day finally came for our visit to the fair when we would see the final touches to the structure. We buzzed with nervous energy as we talked and laughed our way there. To think that a raggedy bunch of dancers from a ballroom had risen to having our very own theater, to display what we had created ourselves!

Approaching the fair was an overwhelming moment.

The last time we were there it had been only bare ground.
The first thing that we saw was the long straight structure,
that held a restaurant from which you could see all over the
fair. Then we saw the globe of the world, it was outstand-
ing! We drove along to the parking lot and piled out of the
cars, we couldn't wait to see the Savoy.

We saw the long, large structure with the name Savoy
running up the side. There were enormous columns that
had life-size pictures of the dancers and our names. As we
entered the building our hearts were in our mouths. We
walked in slowly, and as we did, our enthusiasm hit the
floor. It was not a ballroom, it was a theater, and a tacky
theater at that. The atmosphere was gloomy and cold, the
seating was on plain benches, and the stage was bare and
uninteresting. The set was nothing more than a cheap,
papier-mâche looking prop that somewhat resembled a
bush—this was supposed to represent the jungle and our
roots. The bandstand was in the background and was lit
with the name of the band. The dressing rooms held unpainted
furniture, just some dressing tables with make-up lights.

We were terribly disappointed. Whitey pretended that
everything was fine and went on like it was the greatest
place in the world to work. Still, you could see the disappointment in his face too, and the worst was yet to come.

The working schedule was brutal. We had understood
that there were to be two dance groups working, just as
there were to be two different bands. The musicians, who
had a strong union, had an ideal schedule; Fess William's
band played the day show and Teddy Hill's the evening.
The dancers were to perform every show. The shows,
nearly an hour long, started every hour on the hour from

"The drawing was nothing like the real thing. The building looked something like this on the outside, but on the inside it was cardboard and wooden benches."

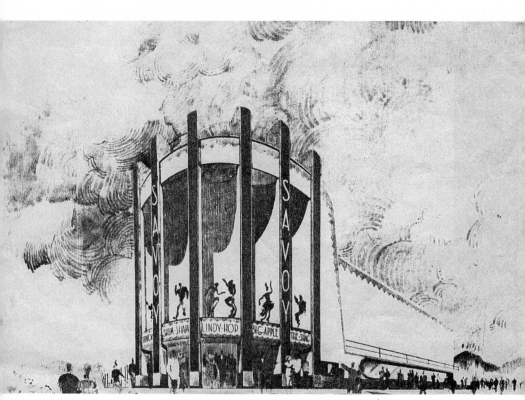

The artist's concept drawing of the Savoy pavilion at the 1939 World's Fair.

noon until six in the evening. Then the night shows started up at seven and went to midnight week nights and two A.M. weekends. We were in a carnival.

Opening day at the fair was a big event, all Savoy personnel were on hand for our opening. After the first show we were applauded, and it was said that we were a great thing for the fair, that we made the fair swing. We were all congratulating ourselves on having gone through with it in spite of the disappointment. After all, we were working every day and getting paid, and that was important. We all agreed that Whitey was some kind of genius. However, by the time the evening rolled around and we had done six shows and had six more to go, our attitudes began to change. We were completely exhausted. I was so tired by the end of the night that I couldn't move anything but my eyelids. Everything ached; my feet felt like biscuits. To think, this would be the schedule for the next six months!

This schedule was unrealistic without two sets of dancers, but Whitey only had one top team available in New York. We were what the public expected, and Whitey always gave the public what it expected. We were the talk of the fair, and we were the only all-black group there. Predictably, tension grew between the dancers, and there were many arguments. It was difficult to understand why Whitey would let us work like that, but we didn't challenge him. We questioned ourselves: Why didn't we back out and insist he get another group? I guess we knew we were all he had at the time.

With youth on our side we endured somehow, but the bickering and exhaustion never let up. I was in charge of the dancers backstage, and Whitey gave me Benny, one of his henchman, to back me up whenever there was a difficult decision to be made. One of my main concerns was appointing dancers to bally—to bally-hoo the show. This is where it became a carnival. The fair exhibits had to compete for business, and this was accomplished by a barker, outside the pavilion who had a spiel for the customers. While he did the spiel, a couple would dance to let people know what was going on inside. This was degrading—the dancers felt they had risen above this kind of exhibition. Eventually we brought in a couple of new dancers solely for this purpose; and the late comers to the show would inherit this job. Our barker was Johnny Vigal, a holdover from the straight days at the Apollo Theater. He would spiel to the public, the dancers would perform their routine, and the people would come.

Business wasn't bad during the day, but it was better at night. The show opened with drums, tom-toms, to set the mood. Our drummers were the best. We had Motorboat and Stewbeef, drummers from the Cotton Club show who could be heard all the way through. Then the African princess would make her entrance, Tanya. She was supposed to be an authentic representation of our roots, but as far as we could see, she looked like a regular shake dancer, and we doubted she'd ever seen Africa!

LeRoy and Little Bea, formerly of the Shorty Snowden Trio, performed the demonstration of the origin of the Cakewalk. After LeRoy would do his strutting Cakewalk, came the Lindy Hop. This was the introduction of a new dance that was nothing short of sensational. It was called Mutiny. Whitey had staged this in the ballroom and we unveiled it at the fair. The staging of Mutiny was the climax of the air steps that we had developed over the past couple

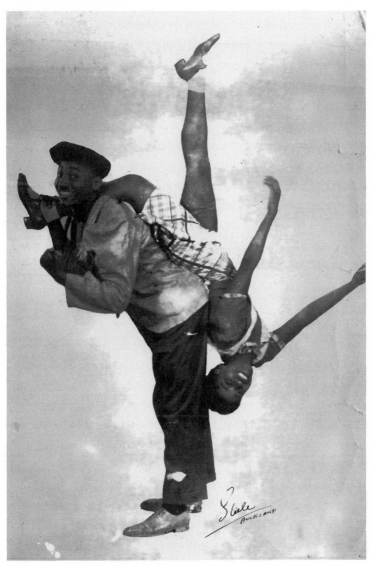

*Frankie Manning and Lucille Middleton in the
Hollywood Hotel Revue in Australia.*

years. This time Whitey had us do our steps together. A team would swing-out from the left side of the stage and another team would swing-out from the right. We would cross each other during the two swings. As the first couple did the step, one did an over-the-head and another an over-the-back, which led to a guy and a gal meeting center stage. The guy would take the gal and pull her between his legs; she would slide on her backside to the guy in the corner, where he would straddle her, pick her up, and throw her over his head. As this unfolded, the other couples would begin their routine. It all happened so fast, the audience didn't know who to watch. It was breathtaking. It got the results Whitey was expecting. The one thing that kept our spirits up while we were working hard as hell was the invigorating response from the public.

The 1939 World's Fair featured a new phenomenon; television. One day, Whitey chose George Greenwich and me to go over to the television exhibit. It was to be a first telecast, and we had no idea what to expect. We had heard about television, but none of us had sets ourselves so it was with a matter-of-fact attitude that we went over to the studio. When we got there we saw that it really wasn't a studio at all, but an outdoor set with one camera and a very small dance space. I was not enthused; I felt I was working hard enough at the fair, and I did not welcome extra work, especially for free.

We were introduced to George Jessel, the host of the show. His face was loaded with makeup; he even wore eye shadow, and his face was pasty white. He asked us our names and we replied.

"We're George and Norma."

"That's great" he said, "I'm a George and Norma too,"

referring to his wife at the time, Norma Talmadge. When he called us to dance, George and I gave a scaled down version of what we did at the Savoy. There wasn't an audience, so we finished to silence. Whitey rushed us back to the Savoy exhibit to do our evening show. The broadcast was rather uneventful, but the Lindy Hop was the first dance to be presented on television.

With our relentless schedule, dancers were getting hurt every show. One night an ambulance had to come for the injured dancers. Mr. Gale's brother was a doctor, and he came out to see us. He came backstage and after examining us, he told his brother that the work was too stressful; he advised closing the exhibit. This didn't hurt our feelings at all. I, for one, completely agreed. After three months, the decision was made to close the exhibit, and we packed up our things and closed the last weekend in June.

Our illusions shattered, and our bodies and spirits exhausted, we could only welcome the return to the Savoy Ballroom for peace and escape.

Whitey already had new plans for us. The *Hot Mikado* was going to the World's Fair. It was to be the first Broadway show to ever play a fair. The theater was called The Music Hall, and the great Bill Robinson would be coming along as the star. Whitey picked his best dancers for the show. This time he would have the giants of the dance. Frankie had just returned from Australia, and with the group from the Savoy exhibit available, he had his top teams to open the show. He added George and me, with Frankie and Lucille, Al Minns and Mildred, and Gladys and Shorty. What appeared to be a disaster wound up back at the top. Whitey bounced back bigger than ever.

While at the fair, Whitey got into a tiff over money with Mike Todd. He was promised a raise if the show was a hit, and evidently Mike Todd reneged on his promise. One day when we arrived at the theater to do the matinée, Whitey sent word down that we were to get dressed, but not go on stage. As usual, we did not question orders.

Our number in the first act was crucial to the production. No one could replace us. We were the show stoppers here. The show began on time, and everything went as it was supposed to go. When the "Three Little Maids" number started and the Lindy Hoppers were to make their appearance, there was a big empty space on stage. The music was playing and everyone stood around, there were no Lindy Hoppers to be seen. We were in the dressing room and heard our cue, but no one said anything. We knew in a few minutes all hell was going to break loose, but we just sat there. Bill Robinson came out of his dressing room and I heard him say to someone outside, "Those kids are just doing what Whitey told them to do." He came into our dressing room and asked us about it. We shook our heads, afraid to say anything or go against Whitey.

Robinson went outside and said loudly, "I want this mess cleared up before the night performance." Whitey was nowhere to be found, we hadn't seen him all day. We understood that when the two of them met in Mike Todd's office, it was like two tigers meeting. Todd didn't know he was meeting with one of the toughest street fighters in show business, but Todd was no pussy cat either. Todd was so upset with Whitey that he picked up a telephone and threw it at Whitey's head. Whitey ducked, and the phone missed him. Somehow they settled their differences and

Whitey got his raise. We didn't. But he sent word to us that the boycott was over. That night when the "Three Little Maids" number came on, the Lindy Hoppers were on the stage and again stopped the show cold. Like Bill Robinson said, "The Lindy Hoppers take care of the first act, I take care of the second."

Nineteen thirty-nine was a big year for Whitey and for Swing. Everybody and everything was swinging. Another classic was to be swung, *A Midsummer Night's Dream*, and it would open at the Center Theater in New York. It would be the biggest show attempted in a theater. It was to have the biggest cast on Broadway and quite an impressive cast it was. The show had a young Dorothy McGuire in the role of the ill-fated lover as well as Louis Armstrong, Maxine Sullivan, Juan Hernandez, Benny Goodman and his quintet, Don Vorhees' twenty-six piece orchestra in the pit, and Butterfly McQueen was Puck. Agnes DeMille did the choreography, and the sets were designed by Walt Disney. Whitey had twenty-four Lindy Hoppers working in the show, the largest number he ever had in one show at the same time. He was the Lindy Hop choreographer. He was riding high, mixing with the greats. He had his own private dressing room and was consulted on all production matters; he was Mr. Big, and indeed he acted the part. We were treated like stars too. It was plush all the way, a far cry from the working conditions at the Savoy of the World's Fair. We were happy as larks, the theater was beautiful, the working conditions ideal. We would perform eight shows a week and have a day off. Even the rehearsals were pleasant. Whitey had a very happy group this time.

Opening night was so exciting. We had a big number in

the second act which opened with Goodman playing a number. The applause seemed to go on forever. Maxine Sullivan was Titania, and we were her little animals in the forest. Bill Bailey had a great Bee's number with the choir singing a cappella with a swinging rhythmic beat. Louis Armstrong was Bottom, the one who's head turns into a jackass's. Mugsy Spanier was on one side of the band shell with his quintet swinging on the growl horn, and on the other side was Benny Goodman, with Lionel Hampton on the vibes, Fletcher Henderson on piano, and Charlie Christian on guitar. Everything in the show was fabulous. Maxine had a microphone, since her voice was very soft and would have been lost without one; they built the mike to look like a snake coming out of the stage. The Deep River Boys were the giant trees that stood in the forest. Whitey had one group of us in the trees and another suspended over the stage. In spite of all this, *Swingin' the Dream* didn't make it. We were devastated by the opening-night reviews. Shows like this are usually blockbusters or complete catastrophes. Some critics said it was a mishmash of Swing and Shakespeare. The lovers were white, and all other members of the cast outside of band members were black. The only thing that outlasted it was the song by Max Gordon "Darn that Dream," recorded by Louis Armstrong and Billie Holiday. The notices were posted for the closing, and the final show was performed amongst a lot of tears and heartbreak. We slowly packed up our things, said our goodbyes, and started uptown, back to the Savoy.

Soon more work came our way. Olsen and Johnson were preparing to do a Broadway-bound show called *Hellzapoppin'*, and we were picked to be its dance act.

We began rehearsals right after *Swingin' the Dream* closed. The show opened in Boston's Schubert Theater. We were to do three weeks there, then come to New York. To us it was a strange show. It wasn't rehearsed like most other shows but was put together with incidents that happened along the way. Olsen and Johnson had always carried their own show, and this was an extension of that show. Comedy teams were riding the wave of Abbott and Costello's popularity. Olsen and Johnson had the wonderful Marty May as the comic playing the violin. The show was a zany type of production. The opening included the entire cast walking across the stage with billboards, throwing pants to the audience, and a film of Amos and Andy (the white ones blacked up) doing a commercial.

Our cue to enter the stage was Andy saying, "As sure as little acorns grow, you can't go wrong with an Olsen and Johnson show!" Then shotguns would go off. They would shoot a double barrel shotgun into a big trash can, and it made a huge explosive sound. Sometimes the backstage of an Olsen and Johnson show felt like a battlefield. I wouldn't come down the stairs until after those guns were fired, it was too nerve wracking.

This show, as well, got very bad reviews. Of course, everything was done to keep it going, and their craziness kept the show alive. The first part of the show to be dropped was our act, not unusual for a show that has to be cut down to stay open. We did the first three weeks before getting the notice, along with other expendable members of the cast. As always, we immediately returned to the Savoy.

"Tiny, who weighed in at something like 400 pounds, did a novelty act."

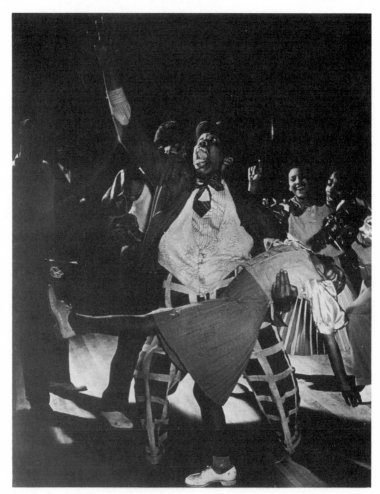

Tiny Bunch and Wilda Crawford at the Harlem Opera House.

Hollywood Calls

Within five years, Whitey had taken the Lindy Hop from a dance hall activity to the biggest venues in show business. From his start as a dancing waiter at Baron Wilkins' Club, Whitey went to the Savoy as a bouncer and, later, floor manager, and from there directly to top dance-director in Harlem. He was an effective organizer, and he knew dancers. He always found dancers who looked like they were enjoying themselves, who had a spark. His dance was the top of the day, and he looked down on all the others. He felt that the dance belonged to him and that he would take his dancers to the top of the heap. He had bettered the Shorty Snowden group, who no longer came to the ball-room. They were much older than Whitey's dancers who were young, bright, fast, and flying high.

Unquestionably Whitey loved his dancers, but he wanted to keep them as they were; he didn't want them to grow. He felt that if he paid them too well they would go out on their own. He did not allow his dancers to take jobs without his consent. If they were called to take a job and the offer did not go through him, they were not to accept it. He demanded loyalty from his dancers, blind loyalty, and his code was a strict one. We danced when and where he told us to or we didn't dance.

In a fight, Whitey resorted to hype. He became the street

thug, the guy who intimidated and controlled the lives of those who came to the Savoy. He had a lot of back-up. His organization had some heavyweight guys to support him in anything he did in the ballroom. His right-hand man in the ballroom was Clyde "Brownie" Brown. Brownie would travel with us when Whitey wasn't available. In the ballroom he had taken over the Saturday night Lindy Hop Contest. Whenever we were in town on a Saturday night we had to dance in the contest, and if we were in town for a Harvest Moon Ball, we were expected to be in that contest as well.

Competition dancing was the life blood of the Lindy and the main source of Whitey's new recruits. He always watched the dancers at the ballroom, he always knew when a dancer in a contest was ready to go to work. When he wasn't there, Brownie was his eyes and ears, always keeping him informed.

One week when Whitey was out of town a job came up with Ethel Waters. Although Whitey was not there to make the deal, a splintered group took the job. Miss Waters knew what dancers she wanted since she had already used them in her review. She called upon Willamae and Snooky to put together a group to play a date in Boston with her. She made them a really good offer.

One sunny afternoon a bunch of us were gathered in the ballroom. Whitey had just returned to Harlem, and everyone was buzzing about the group that did the job with Ethel Waters. Whitey knew he had to do something to make an impression on the rest of us. We all sat waiting, full of nervous anxiety.

Snooky was Whitey's special dancer. He was more

furious with Snooky than the rest of the group, because he
felt Snooky was his own personal property. He had brought
him up from a raggedy, no-shoes, hole-in-the-pants kid.
That day, as he entered the ballroom, Snooky was wearing a
riding outfit, with bright shiny boots. His hair was slicked
down and he was carrying an Australian swagger stick, he
made quite an impression.

He walked in nonchalantly, as if nothing had happened.
Whitey's face was purple, the veins in his neck looked like
they were ready to burst. A group of us were sitting in the
booth as Snooky walked over.

"Hey man, what's up?"

"Nothing but the rent," someone answered.

Snooky looked over at Whitey and said, "Hey Mac."

Whitey approached Snooky and told him to follow him.
They walked down the ballroom to the 140th Street side
with Brownie and a few of his henchmen. It was difficult to
see what was going on at the end of the ballroom. We
heard a noise like someone was being hit.

Words were being passed, "You son of a bitch, after all
I've done for you!"

Whitey struck Snooky again, and Snooky hit the ground,
pleading to not be hit again.

"You punk, get up and fight like a man!" Nothing made
Whitey madder than a man who wouldn't fight, even if he
was getting beaten. Snooky just lay there crying. Whitey
wanted to kill him. But even he couldn't fight a man who
wouldn't hit back, so he called Snooky all kinds of names
while he laid there, looking like a scared kid. Snooky knew
better than to try taking on Whitey.

When Ethel Waters had called Willamae to put a group

together, she knew what she was doing. She knew that Willamae was the most knowledgeable of the girls, because she had taken her under her wing and helped her to see that Whitey was cheating us while we had been on the road with her.

Whitey felt that Willamae had talked Snooky into disobeying his orders. Later that night, after his encounter with Snooky, Willamae came into the ballroom. I knew it was going to be interesting, and wondered how he would handle Willamae since he was convinced that she was the ringleader. She came in with her husband Billy, and she didn't let Whitey frighten her. He wouldn't have dared to hit Willamae as he had Snooky. He knew Willamae had two strong men behind her, and Whitey couldn't afford to alienate Frankie and Billy. Willamae was as stunning as ever. She was an exceptionally good dresser and looked great in whatever she wore. She and Whitey were sitting in the booth; Frankie and Billy were standing nearby.

Whitey was not a stupid man, and he would not do anything to jeopardize his best act. He knew Willamae was the key to keeping the peace, and he was forced to work it through with her. You could always tell when Whitey was on the defensive, he had a way of dropping his bottom lip.

He looked at Willamae with tears in his eyes, asking how she could do this to him. As if all the wrong had been done to him, after all he had done for his dancers. Didn't he put them before everyone, including his wife and his daughter Herberta? Whitey really knew how to turn it on, the difference was that now we all knew him far too well, and none of his sympathetic funk phased us anymore. Instead, it made us laugh. We had been with Whitey from the beginning, we lived with him, we rode in cars with him, we had

seen him at his worst and at his best. He could no longer
suck us in. We were a little wiser now, and we knew we
needed to start making money before we were too old to
dance. You don't have many years as a dancer, and it was
time we started earning some money. It always amazed me
that while Whitey was a very successful man, without us, he
was nowhere.

I had a big argument with Whitey about bringing in
ringers. This particular night we were sitting in the booth in
the ballroom. There was a lull, and we were between
bookings. The question of sending a new group to the
Harvest Moon Ball arose. Most of our teams had already
been in one, or more, of the contests, and he didn't want
the same faces for this one. He wanted Brownie to recruit
new dancers. The Saturday night Lindy contest was still
running, still popular with the Savoy clientele. I felt that
those of us who had been working steadily shouldn't have
to dance in the Saturday night contest, and told him so. He
said, "You never get too big to dance in a contest. That's
the way you started here, and don't you forget it."

That night while watching the contest, a new team went
out and practically did Frankie's routine. I was mad as hell
and looked at Whitey. "How long are you going to let
dancers do our routines? It just doesn't make sense, perfect-
ing a routine and then letting a third-rate dance team copy
it. Wouldn't it be better to keep the top dancing confined
to us, and stop sending ringers in?"

Whitey insisted that those jobs weren't important ones, and
that our group and theirs would never be on the same bill.

"But that's not keepin' our stuff original," I said. He just
walked away, without so much as an argument. I knew why

he was doing it, Whitey had become very greedy. He was making money, and the purity of the dance was not his main interest. He was a man who saw something that he had helped create and that had such instant success, he was afraid it would get away from him. He reacted by grabbing everything in sight. If a job came up and the producers wanted us and we were not available, he would send someone else.

This practice backfired and resulted in Lindy Hop teams springing up everywhere. We felt we would've been making money if he had contained the acts. After working to become the best act, it hurt to see our routines copied. We argued about this regularly.

The groups were demanding more money, and more were taking jobs without consulting Whitey. A group of Lindy Hoppers who were appearing at a club in Harlem, were met by Whitey at the stage door and beaten up. This group decided to do something about it. They signed a complaint with the district attorney and a complaint warrant was issued for Whitey to appear at a special hearing about the allegations made about him.

We were sitting with Whitey in his car when the *Amsterdam News* brought out an extra. The news kids were yelling, "Read all about the Lindy Hop probe!" "Whitey called to testify about dancer beatings!"

Whitey heard them and rushed to get a copy. Talk about hitting the paper; there it was in print that Whitey was intimidating the dancers, that if they didn't dance for him, they were beaten up. In the paper it looked awful, but Whitey felt that what he had done was right, and he simply had been protecting what he had built.

If he had just concentrated on us, this wouldn't have happened. What could he expect when he kept giving other dancers our routines? As soon as they learned to do a couple of swing-outs they went off and got their own jobs. The news in the paper proved to be a tempest in a teapot. However, it was enough to make Whitey return his full attention to his main dancers, and he put together his top foursome to represent him.

The 1940 Harvest Moon Ball was coming up and Whitey wanted Frankie to be in the contest. He also wanted Billy Ricker and me to compete. This would be our last Harvest Moon Ball.

This time Frankie danced with Ann Johnson, and they developed a Mutiny routine that was sensational. It combined a series of flash steps, each step catapulting them into the next. This was where the Lindy Hop had come since 1935 and the first Harvest Moon Ball in which we were told to keep both feet on the floor, and to stay with our partners at all times. Everything had changed, the judges had put the Lindy into its own category, and most of the ballroom rules no longer applied to it. This time out the routines were to be three minutes long with no holds barred. Frankie and Billy worked out their routines in the Saturday night contest at the Savoy. We had a few shows under our belts by now, and we approached the ball with a lot of skill and experience.

This was Frankie's third Harvest Moon Ball and my fourth. The preliminaries were held at the Savoy and the place was packed to the rafters. Everybody was there, rooting for their favorite team. Tops and Wilda were a real smooth dance team and were the hit of the contest. Also dancing were Thomas Lee and Wilda Crawford, they were one of the new teams to catch Whitey's eye. They didn't do many air steps. Instead they relied on a lot of smooth footwork, and they were good.

The big night at the Garden, Ed Sullivan was to be the emcee and the winners would appear in his *Toast of the Town Revue* at the Loew's State Theater.

In preparation we began working out in a gym. Whitey had us practice to a three minute record, dancing straight through. Dancing at a fast pace for three minutes takes conditioning, and we needed to build up our lung power. The first time we danced in the contest we got so tired our teeth felt like they were falling out, our arms got limp, and our lungs felt like they were going to burst! This time we would be better prepared. Our rehearsals were grueling, but we managed to have a good time with it. We had a lot of confidence and knew it wasn't a life and death situation. We knew that Tops could win, even though Frankie and Billy had a good chance as well. Whitey knew that one of us would win, and he hoped it would be Frankie, since he thought that this should be Frankie's last ball. That night at the Garden, Frankie and Billy had the misfortune of dancing at the same time and sharing the points pretty evenly, whereas Tops, who danced first, scored heavily. Tops and Wilda took first prize, Frankie and Ann came in second, and Billy and I, third. After seeing the three winning teams up there at the same time, Ed Sullivan did something never done before or since. He announced to the Garden crowd that he was taking all three winners in the Lindy division to his *Toast of the Town Revue*.

The *Toast of the Town Revue* opened at the Loew's State

Theater after the Harvest Moon Ball. The presentation
starred the winners of the Harvest Moon Ball, and the
dancers were presented doing their routines. First the Fox
Trot, then the Waltz, the Tango, the Collegiate Shag, then
the Rhumba, next the all-around champions, and, finally,
he brought the Harlem dancers on with the Lindy. Opening
day, Billy and I opened the Lindy sequence, then Frankie
and Ann. Then he introduced Tops and Wilda as the champions. The results were not what Sullivan had expected, so the
next show he introduced the champions first, then Billy and
me, then Mr. Lindy Hop himself, Frank Manning, and Ann
Johnson. It was sensational. It made the closing of the *Toast
of the Town Revue* the talk of the town. It was considered
the best Harvest Moon that played the theater. Ed Sullivan
boasted of taking the best of the dancers, and he had proven
himself right to have done something different.

Shortly after our performance at Loew's State,
Hellzapoppin' made a second appearance in our careers.
Although our time with *Hellzapoppin'* had been short, it had
gone on to have many lives. Olsen and Johnson had in-
vested in some high powered publicity. They brought
Walter Winchell to Boston after we left the show, and his
endorsement changed things. He sent *Hellzapoppin'* an
"orchid" which was his blessing. *Hellzapoppin'* came to the
Winter Garden in New York and had a good run. It was
timely, especially for the servicemen who came to New
York. Olsen dedicated his shows to them, which meant
standing room only every show. We had been disappointed
not to be part of its success on Broadway, and thrilled to
return when Olsen and Johnson decided to film
Hellzapoppin', and we were the first act to be called back.

When Whitey got the call from Hollywood he knew he would have to deal with the Lindy Hoppers on a different basis than that of the past. We were more mature, and the deal was going to be different. He couldn't send the ringers, this time he needed his top dancers. The last picture he made he knew he had blundered. He had been called out to do the Judy Garland film, *Everybody Sing!* During the shooting he got into a tiff with the director, and the sequence was cut. He knew he could not make this mistake again, and he wouldn't be going out with the dancers. We were to be supervised by Frankie. He called Mickey and Downes, Billy and me, Al Minns and Willamae Ricker, and Frankie and Ann. We were the foursome he was going to deal with.

Every one of us had argued with Whitey about money at one time or another, and now, we made some demands. We were to travel in style, on a train; no car, no bus. We were to be paid per diem during our stay as well as have our hotel bill paid, plus what we got for the movie. Shooting was scheduled to take two weeks, so we were to receive two weeks salary, plus all expenses. This was very difficult for Whitey. Finally, we would be taking in the money that was meant for us. Whitey would still get his commission, we never felt he shouldn't; we simply wanted our fair share. We were very happy with the deal and felt we had finally accomplished something. We should have known that Whitey would have something up his sleeve, but at the time we were very content with the arrangements.

Leaving for the Coast we took a train to Chicago, where we picked up the *El Capitan* which had sleepers all the way to L.A. When we boarded, we met with the steward and

"This was the ultimate dance group."

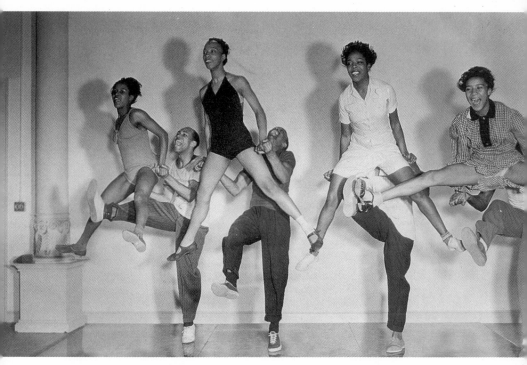

Mickey Sayles and William Downes, Norma Miller and Billy Ricker,
Willamae Ricker and Al Minns, and Ann Johnson and Frankie Manning
(left to right) *rehearsing on the* Hellzzapoppin' *set at Universal Studios*
in 1941.

told him that we would not need to have the beds folded up every day, because we weren't going to get out of bed the whole trip. We intended to sleep all the way West, and that's exactly what we did. We only left the car to eat, then back to the car and sleep; welcome sleep.

Arriving in Los Angeles, we checked into our favorite hotel, the Torrence Hotel at 54th Street and Central Avenue. We were excited to be seeing Mrs. Torrence and her daughter, Lena, again, and they were happy to see us.

We needed a car to go back and forth to the studio, so Lena became our chauffeur. When we arrived at the studio, Olsen and Johnson gave us the star treatment and drove us around the studios in a limo, introducing us to the stars and all the studio heads. It really was grand. *Hellzapoppin'* came to Hollywood with a good track record. It had broken all records on Broadway, and now they wanted to feature our dance in the movie.

Then we were introduced to our choreographer, Nick Castle. This was the first time we had worked with a top Hollywood dance director. We were used to hard work, and the early hours didn't bother us; we could dance at the crack of dawn. We were conditioned to dance on cue. As we walked into the studio, Nick Castle was already there. Ours was a large sound stage, wide and spacious. He came toward us and introduced himself, but we knew who he was from his reputation. Every black dancer who could do a time step knew Nick Castle from his fantastic work with the Nicholas Brothers. There wasn't a black dancer in the country who didn't want to work with Nick Castle. The admiration was mutual because he knew us by reputation as well. Of course, he'd never done any work with the Lindy, but Nick felt that it was a challenge, and if anyone could choreograph jazz it was Nick. We got a chance to talk with him about the great number the Nicholas Brothers did in *Orchestra Wives* and then *Down Argentine Way*, two great classic pictures for the dancers. We knew that here was a guy who understood Swing.

He had just choreographed *Jump for Joy* which was at the Mayan Theater and starred Duke Ellington. He took us to see the show, and told us he thought it lacked a Lindy sequence. Unfortunately, as it turned out, the show didn't run long enough for the addition.

There was one performer that I noticed in particular, he had the most amazing voice. When he spoke it seemed to fill the entire theater, it had me mesmerized. After the show we went back to our hotel. It was late, and we had a long day of shooting ahead of us.

The next night we went to the Club Alabam on Central Avenue where we had performed during our first visit to the Coast. We enjoyed spending our evenings there, we would perform a bit and then just hang out with our new found friends, the West Coast Lindy Hoppers.

That night I was sitting at a table with Ann, we were taking a break from the action when I was amazed to see several *Jump for Joy* cast members walk in. And who was with them but the man with the voice! I elbowed Ann and pointed him out to her. I wanted to walk over to him and introduce myself, but instead I decided to get his attention another way.

I grabbed Frankie and went out on the floor. I really turned it on, I wanted to be sure he'd notice me. As we danced I kept looking over at the actor, making eye contact with him. When the number was over Frankie asked me to dance one more. I told him I was ready to have a seat, and I would send Ann out.

I went back to the table and asked Ann to go out and dance with Frankie. She obliged, leaving me at the table alone. It was exactly what I had hoped for, because my display had worked. The actor approached me and asked if I'd like to dance.

"No thanks," I said. "It's been a long day. I need to sit a few out."

"I saw you dance just now, you're very good. Are you here with anyone in particular?"

"No, there's a bunch of us here. We're all in the same dance group, we're here to do a movie. We're from Harlem. We're doing *Hellzapoppin'* with Olsen and Johnson, we've worked with them before so they called us to do this movie . . ." I was running on.

"That's very interesting. Do you mind if I sit with you?" he said with that incredible voice.

"Suit yourself," I said coolly, regaining my composure.

He sat down and introduced himself, "I'm Roy Glenn. What's your name?"

"My name is Norma, I saw you last night."

"Last night? I didn't see you here last night."

"Not here, in the show. We came over to the Mayan, our whole group. We're working with Nick Castle and he took us to see the show. I saw you perform."

"Good, how did you like it?"

"We liked it fine. I love the Duke."

We began talking about the show . . . his career . . . my career. The rest of my group was impatient to get back to

162

the hotel, I wanted to stay and talk . . . forever. However, we had another early morning coming up, and I knew it was time to go. I told Roy I enjoyed talking to him, but I had to be leaving. He asked me where we were staying and if he could see me home. I agreed to let him but made it clear it wasn't necessary, I could get there fine by myself.

On the way to the hotel we kept talking, and when we got to the entrance we were still talking. There seemed to be so much to say, but I new what we needed to say was, good night. We finally managed, but thankfully not without a good night kiss and a promise to meet at the Club Alabam the next night.

Life on the set was exciting, the scene we were shooting was the jazz scene with some of the top Duke Ellington sidemen including Ben Webster, Lawrence Carney, Slim and Slam, and C. C. Johnson on drums (tom-toms). The scene jumped from the get-go. It seemed that everything in life was becoming a thrill. Here I was, working in Hollywood, in a big movie, and now I had met a wonderful man. What more could a girl ask for?

That night at the Club Alabam my group arrived early. I was having a good time, but I was very eager for Roy's arrival. When he got there we danced a couple of dances, but we mostly wanted to sit in the corner and talk. We were exchanging life stories. I learned that he had been married and divorced. He was twenty-nine and I was only twenty-one, I told him that I had been dancing on the road since I was fifteen and never had had time for a relationship. Finally Roy suggested we get out of the club and asked me if I knew how to shoot pool. I told him I'd never tried, so he offered to teach me, saying there was a hall just down the street.

163

So, we were off to the pool hall, and it was fun. It was so fun in fact that by the time we were thinking about leaving it was dawn. I couldn't believe that so much time had passed. Boy was I gonna hear it from Frankie! Somehow, it didn't seem so bad though. I had the time of my life, just spending time and of all things, learning to shoot pool.

Roy walked me to the hotel and we quickly said our goodbyes. I snuck off to bed, with only an hour before I had to be up again, but I didn't mind. I felt like I could go days without sleep, all was right with the world.

The next day wrapped up our part in the movie. We were asked to do a "movie short" for the jukebox. We had to shoot the scene at night, outdoors, and it was cold; we had to dance in our coats. The short was called *Cottontail*, and was with Duke Ellington. We were happy as hell when we wrapped it up and we rushed off to the Club Alabam. Our time in Los Angeles was ending.

I had only two more nights to spend time with Roy. We had grown very close, and I couldn't stand the thought of leaving. He felt the same, and we decided that I should return to live in Los Angeles as soon as I could wrap up business in New York.

Frankie was notified that we had to return to New York immediately. Whitey had finally dropped the other shoe: Frankie told us that we would not be paid until we got back to New York. Whitey had our check sent directly to him. Talk about slick!

We had no choice, we had to go back. Frankie was strangely quiet. All he could tell us was, "Mac will talk to you when we get to Oswego."

Oswego? What's in Oswego? Frankie then told us that

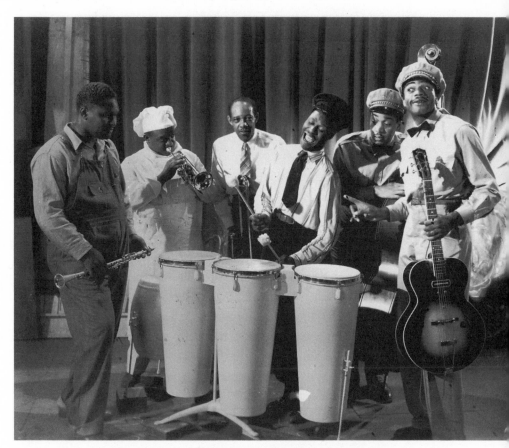

Some of the musicians from Hellzzapoppin': *Slim Gallard, guitar; Slam Stewart, bass; Rex Stuart, trumpet; and C. C. Johnson, drums.*

Whitey had bought a bar and restaurant in Oswego and we
would be going there directly, not even stopping in New
York. It seemed like a lot of changes had been made, and
since Frankie didn't know about all of them yet, it would
be better to let Whitey explain them. Well, there it was.
Nothing more we could do about it. So we packed up and
said our goodbyes.

We said goodbye to Nick first. It had been a great
session, and we felt privileged to have worked with him.
(When *Jump for Joy* was revived some years later, I had the
distinct honor of being asked to assist him.)

The West Coast Lindy Hoppers, who we had spent most
of our evenings with, and Roy all came out to see us off at
Union Station. There were the usual tears and kisses;
goodbyes are always heart breaking when you're young.
We didn't know when we would see each other again.

Roy gave me one last kiss, we held each other tightly for
as long as we could. It could never have been long enough,
I promised I would be back very soon, and then I was on
the train heading back East.

Things were moving so fast for us, everybody wanted us.
We were going from one end of the country to the other,
and it seemed Whitey had more surprises in store. Then
there was talk about the war, and our guys were draft age.
My head was spinning, my heart was overwhelmed with
emotion. I leaned my head back, squeezing my lids as
tightly as I could, but the tears came anyway. Our only
choice was to follow Frankie and do as we were told.

When we reached Oswego, Whitey met us at the train
with his cars and took us to see his new place. Seeing him at
the station was a happy moment, for no matter how dis-

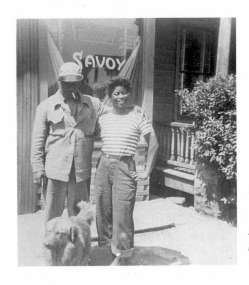

Whitey and Lucille Middleton in front of his bar, the Savoy, in Oswego, New York.

gruntled we felt, we had all missed him. We got into the cars and were taken to Whitey's bar. It had a bar and restaurant in front and living quarters in the back. Whitey was in partnership with Charles Buchanan, and he had the Lindy Hoppers who were not working in a group there with him. His two top girls Lucille Middleton and Pal (Louise Andrews), were in charge of the restaurant, and Whitey took care of the public relations and getting the soldiers to know about the place. This was a very segregated army, and black soldiers had no place to go after hours. Whitey's place became their place away from camp, he had all of the black soldier's business in and around Syracuse. It was a very successful business and a smart move for Whitey, who was already planning his retirement. Now he had only two working groups, and his time was taken up between us and the new business.

When we arrived at the bar we had lunch and finally got

down to the business of being paid. Again, I was terribly disillusioned. We had our salaries cut up; mine looked like Swiss cheese. There were deductions for everything; our hotel bill hadn't been picked up, and we had been charged for all extras. I was so mad at Whitey at that moment that I wished I could just walk away, but I wasn't prepared to do so quite yet.

I could only say, "Just give me what you think I've got coming."

Then Whitey told us the news Frankie had held back: We were to open in Rio in two weeks. The rest of the group seemed delighted, they just mumbled about the rush; but it didn't fit into my plans at all!

"Rio?" I asked, "I'm not going to Rio! I'm going back to L.A., the only reason I came back was to get paid, now I'm gone. What are you talking about, Rio?"

Whitey tried to talk but my mind was made up, and I told him so.

"I don't care what you say Whitey. I can't go and that's that. I've got plans and I'm not gonna break 'em. Nothing you say . . ."

The rest of the group slipped away from the table, and Whitey and I were alone. He scooted closer to me and put his arm across my shoulders. "I already know why you're so upset. Now, what have we talked about so many times in the past? What have I told you from the beginning, about getting involved with men. They're no good for your career. That's not for you Norma, you're better than that."

Frankie, that traitor! "I was only working for you in L.A., and nothing else is your business!" I was fuming, Whitey was calm and paternal.

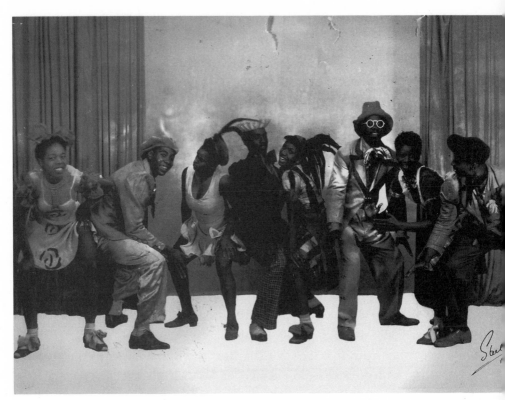

Hollywood Hotel Revue, Australia, 1938.

"Why are you upset with me?" Whitey asked. "You know I'm only telling you this because I care. You're like my own daughter sweetie, I just can't see you throwing away your career over some man. Go to Rio, if you feel the same when you get back, you can go to L.A., with my blessing."

I was defeated. I could not say no to Whitey, I was just too confused and upset to argue any longer. "I know you're right, you always know what's best. Okay Mac, I'll go to Rio. Thanks."

"Anytime, you know I'm here for you."

So there it was, I was going to Rio. We were leaving in such a hurry that we had to get our passports right away. We couldn't wait for the usual couple of weeks to have them mailed. We had to go to Washington, D.C., and apply for them, then wait around for eight hours to pick them up, then immediately to New York to get on the boat for Rio. It all happened so quickly, there was no more time to argue. However, there was enough time for one more change; Downes was drafted. Even Whitey couldn't argue with the U.S. Army. Downes and Mickey would not be going to Rio. So, that left three teams; Frankie and Ann, Al and Willamae, Billy Ricker and me.

Swingin' Down to Rio

We left New York for Rio on a cold winter day,
December 1, 1941. We didn't linger on deck, but
hurried below where we had a small celebration for those
few hearty friends who came to bid us bon voyage. We
hadn't had time to see our friends for the short time we
were in New York, because we were in such a rush to get
off to Rio.

We weren't traveling first class, but the cabins were
comfortable. We looked forward to spending the days ahead
catching up on all the happenings and plain ol' relaxing.

Our second day out, Frankie surprised me with a birthday party in the dining room after dinner, it was my
twenty-second birthday. He had the captain get me a
birthday cake, birthday candles and all. The entire dining
room sang "Happy Birthday" to me. It was wonderful, and
I was really thankful that Frankie cared enough to try and
cheer me up. He knew I was sorely missing Roy.

The spirit of the group was lifting, and I couldn't help
but join them. As we neared Caribbean waters, the weather
began to clear and we emerged from the cabins like moles.
The fresh sea breeze was glorious and the bright sun warm
on the skin.

When the passengers saw the six of us, it wasn't long
before they knew who we were and asked us to perform.

Frankie arranged it, and we did two shows, one for first-class passengers and one for economy class and the crew.

At the ship's first party for the first-class passengers, we danced and were a big hit. We wished we could take that audience with us. After the show, we were invited to the Captain's cabin for cocktails, and we were treated royally. When we said we were swinging down to Rio, we weren't kidding. The trip was a swinger from the sailing date. It was as though everyone went out of their way to make it memorable, anything to make the passengers forget the threat of war.

In this setting it was difficult to believe that a war was going on abroad. Everyone on the ship was trying not to think about it, but there were rumors of war in the air. We hid our fears in humor; it was all so amusing at the time. The ship was white, and every day I noticed that the sailors would touch up the paint. I asked the purser why they were always painting the ship.

Jokingly he answered, "Oh, that's to make us a perfect target."

When we had a fire drill and had to put on life preservers and go to life boat stations, we kidded each other, making jokes about getting torpedoed. Our heads were in the clouds, and we didn't want to see the real world.

"To hell with the war!" we said. "Those bastards over there are always in trouble."

They were endangering our act, and I refused to think about the war one moment more than necessary. I was just a kid.

I'll never forget our arrival. As we neared the Rio harbor, I thought that it had to be the most beautiful harbor in all the world. The magnificent Corcavada stood above all of Rio, from a distance it looked like a giant cross, but as we approached, we could see it was the figure of Jesus, standing over all the people of Rio. It was out of sight. Music began to play the traditional Brazilian Samba, the official music of Brazil. I felt that pulsating rhythm and was overwhelmed, moving to it as naturally as to Swing. The Brazilians have a Swing all their own, but it has the same African roots as American Jazz. Brazilian blacks gave it a Samba beat, and American blacks swung it. The ties were there, and we felt them immediately. Everything about Brazil was swinging.

A representative of the casino met us at the dock to be sure we would have no trouble with taxis or checking into our pension. It wasn't a hotel, but a private home that provided bed and breakfast. Once we were settled, we were taken to the casino. The driver took us along Copacabana Beach where the road winds all the way to the Casino De Urca, a beautiful building on the beach, with an awning all the way to the street. It was just as we anticipated, like a fabulous movie setting. There was nothing in America to compare with this casino. It was on the beach, facing the harbor, and when you stood on the patio looking across the harbor, you had a breathtaking view of the statue of Christ. Rio immediately filled a special place in my heart. It was so full of beauty, and the Brazilians were as good as their city. You could feel their passion for it. It was infectious and enveloped us completely.

Frankie met with the band while we had a chance to explore the casino. We were told politely that we were not to gamble, as the casino profits were paying our salaries. That wasn't a problem for us, we weren't high rollers. It was enough for me just to be there, to be in Rio, listening to Brazilian music. Our first rehearsal we paid particular attention to the music, we had Basie charts.

The Carlos Machado Band was the big band in Rio. It had eighteen musicians with the regular brass and horn section, but the rhythm really made the band. In addition to the drum, it had a tambourine and the big shell with the beads around it, which had a special sound that got a person into Samba. With our Basie charts, our music was considered real Swing music, and the band used our music for their own sets. When the band began to play though, we heard something different. Along with the swing beat that the drummer was playing, we now had an extra set of rhythms that we had never heard before. A Swing dancer has a keen ear for the beat, and we dance to what we hear. Usually, a drummer follows the dancers, but now we had three extra guys doing that. They played the hell out of that music! We knew we were going to have our first great opening outside of the United States. We took to their music as though it were our own.

The Casino De Urca had everything; three big bands, a large chorus line like the Rockettes, and over one hundred band singers. It was something like Las Vegas is today. These girls didn't have to be great singers, but they had to be beautiful. All through the night, while the bands played dance music, a different girl would appear to sing one number with the band. They sang in different languages, most were German girls running away from the war. It seemed like half of Germany had rushed to Brazil. The show had two organ players, who played at intermission while a giant mirrored curtain across the stage unfolded. We were awe struck watching the production. One of those organ players was the great Ethel Smith, who brought the Samba to Hollywood. On that same bill was the Brazilian star Grande Otello, the Sammy Davis, Jr., of Brazil. He was a great entertainer, song writer, and singer, who looked like a little, beautiful monkey. The Casino De Urca was also the home of Carmen Miranda before she went to Hollywood.

Opening night in Rio was an exciting event. We loved Brazil, and Brazil loved us. When we hit the stage with the band, I knew something special was happening. It was wonderful, it was that Samba beat. As each couple finished, we would call out, "Now follow that!" and we'd walk off cockily. The house roared, and the band was swinging like crazy. When we finished, the house went wild, everything else stopped. We bowed and bowed, and, finally, they let us go. We were a smash in Rio. We knew we had found a second home.

We were so thrilled with our opening that the next day Frankie arranged for us to have the cook's tour of Rio. As we were walking to the Rio Brancs, Rio's main drag, we noticed America in the newspaper headline and asked Frankie, who understood the language, what it said.

"America has declared war. Japan bombed Pearl Harbor" he read.

We looked at each other, "What in the hell is a pearl harbor?" And with that we walked on down the street, trying not to think about it. But we were in the war, damn it! Even though we hadn't yet felt its effects, it was happening. With the war would come a lot of changes. It was a strange feeling, being in a foreign country and knowing our own country was at war. At the time it seemed more of an

inconvenience than anything else, but the feeling of being
Americans began to overcome us. I remembered Mama
always making such a point of my being born in America,
but this was the first time it had any real meaning for me.
We realized that the war would affect us directly because
our guys were draft age and would be called to fight. Then
what was going to happen to our act? They had only been
given a three month extension from the draft board.

But what's the point in worrying about the future when
it's out of your hands? "To hell with it," I decided, "right
now we are going great in Rio." Our contract was for six
weeks, and we had return passage tickets already booked. So
we settled in, but when six weeks were over, Frankie told
us we would not be able to leave by ship. The Germans
were bombing everything leaving Brazil, and only oil
tankers were trying to get through. It would not be safe for
us to take a tanker, although sometimes they carried passengers. So, we kept on working. Our options were picked up,
and we dodged the draft board a little longer. Six weeks
became ten months. We played all the casinos in Brazil. We
would do our first show of the evening at the Casino De
Urca, then we would take a cabin cruiser across the harbor
and play a second show at the Casino Icarai.

During our stay in Rio, Orson Wells began filming
Carnival there. The casino was used for a film set during the
day, and Orson Wells sat in the center of the room directing
the film. He had a voice just like Roy's. In fact, the first
time I heard him speak, my heart leaped, and I was sure that
Roy was in the room. After we had been introduced, I
would sit by his side, just to hear him speak. He would talk
to me because I was one of the few people around the set

who spoke English. I could listen to that voice and watch the production all day long.

As things worked out, we were able to stay in Rio for Carnival. We had been told about it since our arrival, and we were looking forward to it. Grande Otello wanted us to be his special guests and see it first hand. Grande was like the Grand Marshall in the parade, and we were right beside him. It was colorful and fun, the costumes were extraordinary. The entire city was dancing in the streets, and we joined right in, having a ball.

We all became good friends with Grande during our stay in Rio. I noticed him putting his head together with Frankie's, and I wondered what they were up to. We soon found out.

Closing night is always special, and all the acts try to do something unique. For us, everything started out the same, until Frankie swung out. Instead of Ann, he had Grande, dressed as a girl in a white flowered dress with a belt around his waist, a ribbon in his hair, and white flat-heeled shoes. When Frankie swung across the stage with Grande, the house stood up. When he threw Otello over his head, he looked like he was walking on air. It was sensational, and typical of Frankie. He could keep a secret better than anyone I knew. It was a complete surprise to us all, and it was a fitting closing night.

Our next engagement was in Mini Gerais, Pampoulia. The Casino Pampoulia, built in the interior of Brazil, was new, and they had to build a road to the casino so you wouldn't have to cut through the jungle with a machete to get there. It had a beautiful glass floor, lit from underneath in differently colored squares. Ours was the first show to play the Casino Pampoulia.

It seemed the further we tried to get away from the war, the more enmeshed we became. Our pension in Rio catered to foreigners. As it happened we found ourselves living with sailors who had been under house arrest for two years, captured with the *Graf Spee*. One morning at breakfast one of them asked Billy, "Do you know that we are Germans?"

Billy shrugged his shoulders and answered, "So what? Your German."

The sailor was surprised, but that broke the ice, and we found ourselves speaking to them when we came down to breakfast and not viewing them as Germans, but as human beings. They were surprised that we didn't hate them, but we had always felt that you couldn't hate someone you didn't know. But war changes things, and it wasn't long before Brazil entered the war.

One day shortly after we arrived in Mini Gerais, we were doing a matinée and decided to go sightseeing on the way to work. We didn't think that this was going to lead to trouble, but as we were standing at a bus stop, a crowd began to gather. Everyone was trying to get on the bus; we gathered our group and began edging closer to the bus. People were becoming impatient and maybe worried that they wouldn't get on or wouldn't get a seat. Suddenly there was pushing and shoving and someone deliberately pushed Willamae. I was in back when I saw Billy reach over and hit someone, then Frankie let loose on a man's nose.

The next thing I knew, we were sitting in jail saying, "Don't get us involved in an international situation!" It seemed like a joke, and we never gave it any more thought than that. We were released from jail and sent to our matinée. It was a good fight, and we had won. Our guys were very protective of us; they were taught always to defend us, and were taught never to put a guy in jeopardy without due cause. This time it was warranted, one of us was attacked, and we responded. It seemed to end there.

When we arrived at the casino, we were the talk of the show, but we laughed it off, and worked the matinée as usual. After the show we went to our hotel, the Hotel Paradise. It was a new hotel; everything was first class. It even had an elegant dining room on the roof. That night when we returned from our long day's work, we had our usual coffee and conversation in the dining room before we went off to bed.

By the next day we had put the incident out of our minds, but that night as we were preparing to leave for work, we heard a lot of people gathering on the street below. We thought it was the theater directly across the street letting out. Billy looked out the window and re-marked that there must be a great picture playing over there because there were sure a lot of people coming out of the theater. Someone knocked at the door. It was the manager, wanting to speak to Frankie. When Frankie came back, he looked very serious. He went to the window and cautiously closed the drape. He got everyone together and told us that the crowd milling about outside had pipes and stones to throw at us. We didn't know that this ordinary street incident had gotten tangled up with politics. A U.S. ambas-sador had signed some kind of agreement related to Sumner Welles's Good Neighbor Policy. The Germans in Brazil were worried about what that would mean for them, so they were instigating Brazilians to embarrass the U.S. and challenge the policy. And there were plenty of Brazilian nationalists who didn't want to see the agreement signed anyway. Our joke about an international incident was becoming a serious worry.

Frankie, Ann, and I were together when we heard the sound of hoof beats. The state had sent the militia to control the crowd. We gathered our things as quickly as possible and went down the elevator, surrounded by police who were trying to shield us from the angry crowd.

Frankie told us, "Everyone grab someone and hold on to him for dear life."

When we got to the lobby the police ordered us to return to our rooms. It was getting ugly. We could hear the crowd shouting at us but we didn't understand what they said. We were astonished that people could turn on us so quickly. Someone had done a bang up job on them, and we felt we were in danger of being lynched.

We were in the hotel room not knowing what to do next, when suddenly Ann, who could sometimes be a very funny chick, broke wind.

Frankie turned around, embarrassed, and said, "Oh, Ann!"

She came back quickly, saying, "Well, haven't you ever heard of the shit being scared out of you?"

We all broke up laughing, it was the perfect tension breaker. That night we didn't go to work, nor did we ever return to the Casino Pampoulia. We were escorted out of town, two in a car, with four secret service people including the driver surrounding us. We were taken to the next town, where we got a train to take us back to Rio. Everyone at the Casino De Urca was glad when we safely returned there.

Orson Wells, in his booming voice, asked us "And how was the fair city of Mini Gerais?"

We all laughed and said, "Never again!"

During most of our ten months in Brazil, our country had been at war and we were just beginning to feel its effects. Frankie announced that he had booked us on flights from Rio to Miami, and we would be leaving in two shifts. Al, Ann, and I would take a flight one day, and Willamae, Billy, and Frankie would follow two days later. We all would meet again in Miami. Flights were hard to come by, and this was the best he could do under the circumstances. We were glad, we felt it was about time we returned to the United States. It was the end of an era for us. We knew that when we returned, our guys would be leaving, and we began to think about the future.

All of that would come in time, for now we focused on going home; reality will remain on hold for only so long. It had been great in Rio, and we hated to leave. At least we had learned the Samba, and we would be taking that back home with us. I had been dancing in the Brazilian ball-rooms as much as I could and had learned the dance fairly well. I planned to incorporate it into whatever I decided to do next.

We prepared to leave, and Frankie gave us our instructions. He was a real hero. He took care of our transportation, and he was generous and strong. He never once complained about the way we acted. I never saw him lose his temper. If ever a man fit the phrase, "Keep your head when everyone around you is losing theirs and blaming it on you," it was Frankie. Whitey wasn't there, and Frankie took the blame for whatever went wrong, he never retaliated or tried to blame anyone else. As I look back on those days, I thank him, as I never thanked him before. The Lindy Hop owes Frankie Manning a special award. He kept the dance alive.

We arrived in Miami, Florida in November 1942. It was the first time I had personally experienced the prejudices we had heard about in the South. Black people were completely segregated; I couldn't believe it. Nothing I had experienced prepared me for this. I had known that segregation existed, but it wasn't until I saw it first hand that it became real to me. We had traveled all around the world, had been embraced by countless people who loved us, so to face this in our own country was a real shock. We had been through a lot by now and felt we could adjust to anything. Being international travelers, we were welcomed with open arms by the colored people of Miami. They took us to their main drag, Second Avenue. I had never seen so many black faces in one area in my life, not even in Harlem; after being in a foreign country for so long, we relished them. It was good to hear American voices, even with a southern accent. The strange thing was, the Miami accent sounded almost foreign to us. It took a little getting used to. Being back in America was good enough for me, and I kissed the ground when we arrived. We hadn't gotten back to New York yet, but we would be soon, and at least we were in the States.

People found out who we were, it was a small area, so it didn't take long before they asked us to perform. When Frankie arrived, he took charge as he always did, and he arranged for the folks to see their famous visitors from up North perform.

There was a big show, and we were the stars that

evening. It was a thrill to dance for an American audience, and we took the town by storm. We hadn't lost touch after all. There was a big celebration after the show. In a few days, we left Miami and headed North.

Our last official job with Whitey was a date at the Apollo Theater, with Cootie Williams and Pearl Bailey; it lasted three weeks. We performed at the Apollo in New York, the Howard in Washington, and the Royal Theater in Baltimore. This was the last three weeks we would work together as an act. The draft hung over us like a cloud. The end was near, and we all felt it. Whatever we did would be up to the draft board, and they seemed a little annoyed at our guys for having been given special exemptions from the Army. We girls talked about it often. I didn't feel I wanted to get another partner, the time had come for me to do something on my own. It would be too distressing to lose another partner to the draft.

As we went into rehearsal for the show, nothing was the same. The future was so uncertain that we danced half-heartedly. We played the Apollo, and the crowd's enthusiastic welcome made us feel great about getting back in harness. But then we went to Washington, D.C., where Billy was called to the Army and told to report for duty after the Baltimore show. That clinched my future, my mind was made up for me. My days as a Lindy Hopper were drawing to a close. It had been great; we had been around the world, and now it was time to do something else. Whitey's Lindy Hoppers had a few more dates before Frankie too was called to war.

Moving On

The '40s saw changes in music and dancing. Our act was now disbanded, our guys were all in the Army. The big band sound of Swing was being taken over by the Latin Invasion. The Palladium was drawing the people now. The dancer Frank "Killer Joe" Piro was teaching Afro-Cuban dance there. Everywhere they were doing the Mambo. It was becoming so big that Jimmy Durante was quoted as saying, "Beethoven goofed, he didn't write a Mambo."

In the theaters Katherine Dunham's dancers were the ones to watch with their sensual, primitive style. In October of 1940 they had opened *Cabin in the Sky* with Ethel Waters at the Beck Theater. On the other side, came Agnes DeMille with her 1943 introduction of modern ballet in *Oklahoma*.

I saw Whitey for the last time in the foyer of the Savoy. He was sitting by himself and he seemed so lonely, I felt sad for him. He was used to having a bunch of dancers around him, and seeing Whitey like that made me realize how different things really were. We were so close at one time, but the war seemed to have changed that too.

He greeted me warmly, "Hi kid. How's it going?"

"Fine," I said, "how are you doing?"

"Listen, I've been thinking over an idea I've had for a long time. Now that the guys are gone, why don't you take

"DuNham brought lots of sexuality into dancing. When we saw how she had used caribbean rhythms in cabin in the sky, we knew that dancing had changed forever. The people loved what she was doing."

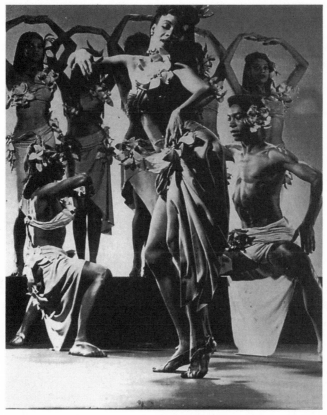

Katherine Dunham dancing to Caribbean rhythms in Cabin in the Sky.

over the new group for me? You've led your own group before, and I'll back you. You could even use your own name, as head of the group."

It was tempting, but it was still just Lindy Hopping. I wanted to move on to other things, I was interested in all kinds of dance, and I didn't want to limit myself to just one style. I wanted to explore the various styles that were making inroads in the dance field such as Katherine Dunham's primitive, native style that was so identified with the Caribbean. Then there was the new modern dance that was being introduced by Martha Graham and Hanya Holm. I wanted to learn these. So I declined. I felt there would never be a better time to make a complete break, and I knew my opportunities were elsewhere.

"Thanks Whitey," I told him, "but I'd rather start all over again with my own ideas of dancing."

He was gracious, he said he was sorry we couldn't get back together, but he wished me the best, and he told me if I ever needed anything I should let him know. I thanked him, and we promised to stay in touch.

As I walked away, I felt downhearted, we had shared so much affection. What I knew about the business, I owed to him. He made us a great act. Through him, we became good, dependable dancers. These were characteristics that would carry all through my life in show business.

With all of the new dancing that was taking place in New York I immediately enrolled in a dancing school. It was called the New Dance Group. The school was on 59th Street, and taught all the modern styles. There was the Hanya Holm style taught by Mary Anthony, The Humphrey-Wideman style taught by Charles Wideman,

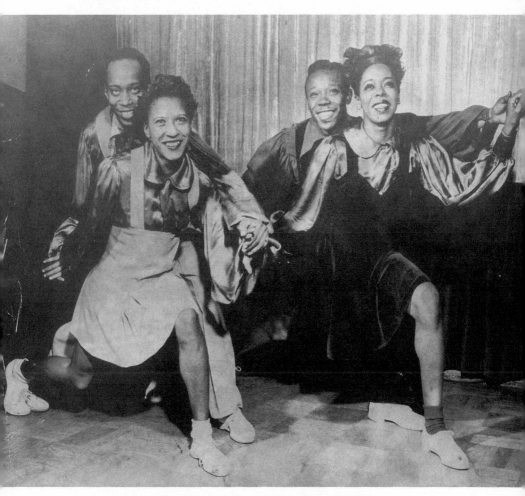

*Leon James and Ann Johnson, Willamae Ricker and Ali
dancing at the Club Delisa in Chicago, 1943.*

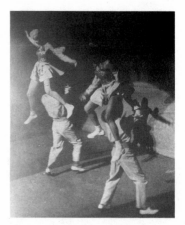

The Congeroos: Helen Daniels and Franking Manning, Willamae Ricker and Ali, circa 1942.

and of course Martha Graham's style, taught by Sophie Maslow. These were the best dance classes in New York, and I took them all.

While attending school I supported myself by working at Small's Paradise where I produced the shows for a year. Between taking classes all day and working at night, my body was taking a beating. The Graham technique was playing havoc with my knees.

In the meantime I became a Broadway gypsy, auditioning for every show that came along. When the casting call for Billy Rose's *Carmen Jones* was announced, I was the first in line. It was a grueling audition, call back after call back. I was among the few who made the final cut. When we received the contracts, I nearly laughed. The salary was unbelievable. I had left Lindy Hopping to better myself, and the salary I was being offered was pathetic! I told Billy Rose what I thought of it. I was making more at Small's Paradise, and I made that clear to him.

He was not happy and told me, "Small's Paradise is a salt mine compared to *Carmen Jones!*"

I told him, "I'll take the salt mine!" and left without looking back. So much for me and Broadway.

Working in Small's Paradise gave me the chance to explore the types of shows I wanted to present. I put out feelers to go on the road, and I was fortunate to be booked right away as a single act, singing and dancing. My first date was in Montreal, Canada. It was strange to me to be working on my own, but I was making money chasing my dream, and that was all that mattered. I worked my way across Canada to the West Coast.

By the time I finished my last date in Canada, I had just enough money to buy a train ticket to Portland, Oregon, where I was to perform next. The train stopped overnight in Seattle.

I was completely broke, I didn't even have enough money for a room for the night, let alone dinner. It was time to come up with a plan. I lugged my baggage into the ladies room and went to work. I freshened up and got dressed in my best; a slick, red, shark skin suit I'd had made in Rio, with a red, dipped hat, plumes and all, and red platform shoes, just like Carmen Miranda's. I returned to the station lobby and perched atop my luggage. I was hungry and I was tired, but I looked good.

I sat fingering my last dime. It was all the money I had in the world, and I wondered what in the hell I was doing there. Before long I was getting looks from men hurrying through the station, one stopped to ask me if I was waiting for a ride.

"No," I told him, "I'm just waiting, period. I'm heading for Portland, and I don't leave until morning."

"I see," he said, "maybe I'll see you at dinner then."

"Not unless I can get dinner with this ten cent piece" I said, holding up the dime.

"You tellin' me that's all the money you got? You travelin' by yourself?"

"That's right."

"What is a young lady like you doin' traveling alone with no money?"

"I'm an entertainer, it don't bother me none. I can take care of myself."

"Well, I'm sure you can. Still it probably wouldn't hurt you to have a good meal tonight, would it?"

"I don't suppose it would."

"I wait tables in the restaurant, I'm gettin' ready to go on shift. Why don't you give me about twenty minutes and go on in, don't order from nobody 'til I get there, and I'll fix you up with some dinner."

I smiled gratefully. "That would be real nice."

I waited half an hour, not wanting to seem overly anxious and then went into the dining room. It was crowded, and I wondered how he would ever find me. I settled into a seat in the corner to wait, the padded chair was much more comfortable than my luggage.

A gentleman who was sitting across the way noticed me and struck up a conversation. We chatted across the aisle, and he asked if he could join me. He seemed nice enough, and I was restless, so I agreed. He told me his name was John and that he was traveling to a new job in Canada, he was in sales. He asked about me, where I was coming from and where I was going. I told him about my recent trek across Canada, and my career, never mentioning the fact that I was broke. He was very interested in the entertainment business and listened intently. When the waiter came to the table I was pleased to see it was my new friend from the lobby. We ordered plenty of food and when the waiter didn't seem put out, I requested wine.

We kept up our conversation, and when the food came I ate ravenously. When the waiter returned to see if there was anything else he could bring us, John asked him to bring both checks. John said he would pay for mine. The waiter smiled, and I was glad that he wouldn't be stuck with my large bill.

We continued talking, when suddenly John realized his train was due to leave. He had to rush and apologized for not walking me to my hotel. I was actually relieved that he was not spending the night in town. I thanked him, and we wished each other good luck. He shook my hand and left the restaurant. My waiter returned to the table when he left.

"So, you had a lot of offers for dinner tonight," he said. "I'm not surprised, a pretty lady like you. Are you meeting him later?"

"No, he's on his way out tonight. Besides, the only thing I got on my mind is sleep."

"So where you stayin' anyway?"

"I guess right here in the station."

"That's no good. You know, there's a place up the street, it's nothing fancy but I could get you a room there real cheap."

"I wasn't kidding when I said all I got is a ten cent piece. No room is that cheap."

"I'll take care of it for you. I got about an hour left to work, why don't I bring you some coffee while you wait, then I'll walk you over."

"Why would you do that for me? You don't even know my name."

"You got a good laugh. Besides, you shouldn't be spendin' all night in this train station, who knows what could happen. By the way, my name is Henry."

I extended my hand, "Pleased to meet you Henry, my name is Norma Miller. A good nights sleep sounds real good, I'll take it."

While I waited for Henry to finish I wondered what he expected in return. An offer like his with no strings attached was unusual, but I decided to deal with it when I had to; for now I needed rest.

Henry returned as soon as he was finished working. Being quite tall and muscular, he picked up all of my belongings himself. We walked to the hotel, chatting. As promised, he got me a room and left. The next morning I was back on the train heading for Portland. I never saw Henry again, but I still remember him with gratitude. Funny how sometimes guardian angels come along.

I completed my dates in Portland and left with enough money to get to L.A. and find work. I was eager to see Roy, so much had happened since I was last in L.A., I wondered what it would be like when I saw him again. I called him as soon as I arrived only to discover that he was in Europe.

When Roy returned and got the message that I was in town he rushed over to see me. We were thrilled to be reunited. Our meeting was not what I expected, but these things never are. The world around us was not all that had changed. As the song says, some things start too hot not to cool down.

We tried to make the relationship work, but that initial connection was lost.

I worked with various dance groups on the West Coast through the war years. I was working in a variety show with Pigmeat Markham at the Lincoln Theater on Central Avenue in 1943, when I got a surprise visit from Frankie Manning. His unit was in L.A., and they came to see the show. All dressed up in their uniforms, they looked so handsome. But, they were only in town for the weekend, so I didn't get to spend much time with him. I had missed Frankie and it made me very happy to see him and know that he was safe, and I was so proud of him. There were many servicemen in our audience as the war plodded on, and we all wondered when it would end.

D-Day, June 6, 1944, our troops crossed the English Channel to invade Normandy. Soon the war in Europe was over, thank God. Meanwhile, our own show went on. The production with Pigmeat was a variety show, like those at the Apollo, a stock job which meant we changed shows every week. He had a big band led by Bardu Ali and a line of girls, which I joined temporarily. The show lasted through the rest of the war years.

We were in the Lincoln Theater on April 12, 1945 when we got the shocking news that Roosevelt was dead. It seemed that he had always been president, and his death only made us more anxious about the war. That damned war was always with us. Harry Truman took office, two atomic bombs were dropped on Japan in August, and at last Japan sued for peace. After all of this horrible destruction, the war was over.

I chose to stay on the West Coast for a while. I was still involved with Roy, and I had the opportunity to produce some shows at the Club Alabam, one of which included Johnny Otis and his fifteen-piece band. Otis was a terrific drummer and an important influence on music. He introduced Little Esther (Phillips) and recorded with the young Etta James. He's white but he always lived black. His music is the real thing. He's a minister now, I believe.

When my schedule allowed, I enjoyed going out and dancing socially, especially at the L.A. Cotton Club where Basie often performed. One night Milton, a good friend of mine, and I caused quite a stir. He was a white feller and a good dancer. Basie was on the stage and we decided to go out and take a few swings on the floor. People were staring at us in an odd way, and we wondered why. It didn't occur to us until later that it was over my being black and his being white. Los Angeles was not accustomed to integrated dancing in 1945. The Savoy was a long way away.

In 1946, Roy got his first break on Broadway, a role in *Anna La Casta*. There was a lot happening on the East Coast at the time, and I felt it was a good time to return to New York. Roy and I packed up and we hit the road in my car, an old La Salle.

When we got there, I found that some of the old gang were dancing again. Frankie had put together The Congeroos, a four-person act with Willamae and Ali, and Ann and himself.

While in New York, I stayed with my mother. Getting jobs was not difficult, I was producing shows and always included my own act. With both of us in the business, my relationship with Roy suffered. His acting career was beginning to take off, and for both of us our careers came first. As much as we loved each other, our relationship was second. We put our marriage plans on hold too many times. Something always seemed to keep us from walking down that aisle. I seemed destined for the single life.

When I got the opportunity to take a show to St. Louis, off I went. I spent the next few years traveling with different shows, never making time for romance. Maybe I liked my independent, spontaneous life too much. I don't recall making a big decision to stay single. I just did.

Not that it was easy to be on my own and responsible for a group of dancers. I had been around and observed what having that responsibility meant day to day; so I had some foundation for being in charge. And I was also lucky to have met some wonderful people in my travels; it seemed as if there was always somebody I could count on for help when trouble hit. Joe Louis stands out as one of the most generous and kind people I have known.

I met Joe Louis just after he became the world champion heavy weight boxer. After his big fight in 1938, he used to come to the Savoy Ballroom, and he always gravitated toward the kids. He was a man with very little education but when he became so famous, he never pretended to be sophisticated nor did he try to get special treatment. Lots of people, when they get big and famous, talk down to people. Sugar Ray Robinson did that, but Joe never did. He had a kind of in-grown sensitivity. So he felt he could be himself around us kids at the Savoy. I remember he like peanuts, ice cream, and movies!

Most of the time money was very tight, and we struggled just to get by. Anytime word that I was in need got to Joe through the grapevine, he would come through. I would get a message at the Hotel Theresa in New York to meet him at Mrs. Fraiser's, a famous eating place for the black elite of the sports world, and he would meet me there, doing whatever he could to help out.

Joe Louis, still champion, retired from boxing on March 1, 1949 and took some time to travel and relax, he enjoyed living big. That same year he and his first wife, Marva Trotter, divorced. My group of dancers and I were performing in Miami, Florida, when we got word that the Champ was in town. At the time Miami was very segregated. We were staying at the Mary Elizabeth Hotel, where all the black entertainment and sports figures crossed paths. We met up with Joe there and were asked to pose for pictures with him for the newspaper. We all obliged, and then one of the newsmen started questioning Joe.

He asked, "So, Mr. Louis, will you be playing any golf while your in town?"

Joe looked at Al Williams of the Step Brothers and asked, "What day do we play?"

Al said, "We play on Wednesday," meaning that Wednesday was the one day that blacks were *allowed* on the course.

Joe looked at the reporter and said, "I'll be playing on Wednesday."

Then he walked away. Now, Joe could have played any day he wanted to. He was offered many privileges that other blacks were not allowed, but he never took advantage of them. He refused to be set apart simply because of his position.

Joe was a magnet for people, and while he was in town

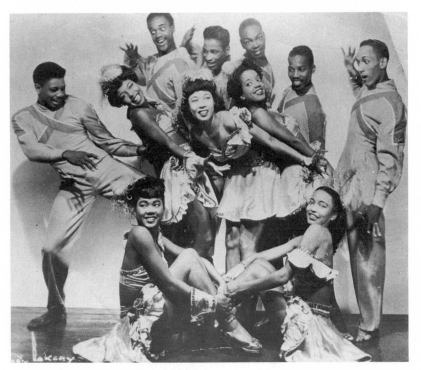

*The original Norma Miller Dancers, circa 1953. Back: Joe Noble,
Frank Kilabrew, and Billy Dotson; middle: Curtis, Geri Gray, "Pudgi,"
Priscilla Rishad, Scotty, and Raymond Scott; front: Leona Laviscont
and Barbara Taylor.*

they came from everywhere. During the same stay in
Miami, Barry Grey, a white, liberal radio personality,
invited Joe to a broadcast from the Fontainebleau Hotel.
But the hotel did not allow blacks. Joe refused, graciously
telling Barry, "I don't go where my people can't go."

When Barry Grey went on the air he tore into Miami
and its racist policies, saying in no uncertain terms that he
had invited the world's heavyweight champion to appear on
his show, but Mr. Louis refused, because the Fontainebleau
did not allow his people to come into their hotel. Barry
Grey, as we say in Swing lingo, "read them."

We had bookings but not a lot of cash, and while in
Miami, we ran out of money. Our entire costume wardrobe
was at the cleaners, and I needed seventy-five dollars to get
it out, but had no resources left and decided to ask Joe for
help. We had a job coming up at the Bill Rivers Club and
would be able to pay him back after the gig. Well, Joe
always had a way of doing things without any fan fare. I was
sitting in the lobby, waiting to hear from him when he
came in with his entourage (he always traveled with an
entourage). He had just come from a ceremony at which
they presented him with a tie. As they walked in, they were
all kidding Joe about the tie and its loud colors.

Poker faced Joe responded in his simple way with words,
"It's free ain't it?"

He came over to me, and when he reached down to
greet me, he dropped the tie into my lap.

"The money is in the tie" he whispered.

I put the tie in my bag so no one would see it. Later I left
the lobby to look inside the tie and sure enough, there was
the money I needed for costumes for the show that night.
Not only did Joe Louis give me the money for the costumes, but he sent word to Bill Rivers that he would make
a personal appearance and allow his name to be used on the
bill with my dancers. We packed the place and were assured

of a paycheck. Joe Louis was a wonderful friend and a fine
human being. My dancers loved him, I loved him.

In these years just after the war I still thought of New York
as my home. I stayed there for some time in 1950. I didn't
see Whitey when I got back, but I heard he was living
upstate in Oswego where he had his business. He died there
that year. I didn't get the news right away, and by the time
I did, he had been buried. I'll always regret missing his
funeral. So much of what connected me to New York was
slipping away.

I went by the Savoy a couple of times, but it wasn't the
same. It didn't hold the fascination it once had. I didn't
know anyone anymore, and it seemed that everyone had
forgotten the Lindy Hoppers. I finally realized that there
was no reason to go back. The doors of the Savoy closed in
1958, and by that time most of the entertainment in Harlem
was gone. All we had left was Small's Paradise on 135th
Street and 7th Avenue and the Baby Grand on 125th Street.

I was living with Mama on 129th Street, on the top of a
six floor walk-up. The streets had become a frightening
place to be after dark. I would go out in the evenings,
knowing I could not return home until daybreak. The clubs
were only open until four A.M., but, fortunately, I knew
most of the owners so I would sit with friends until six A.M.,
when I could return home safely. The junkies were usually
asleep by then. Something terrible was happening to
Harlem; some said it was genocide. The places of entertainment were closing. Taxi drivers were warning their customers that coming uptown to Harlem was too dangerous.

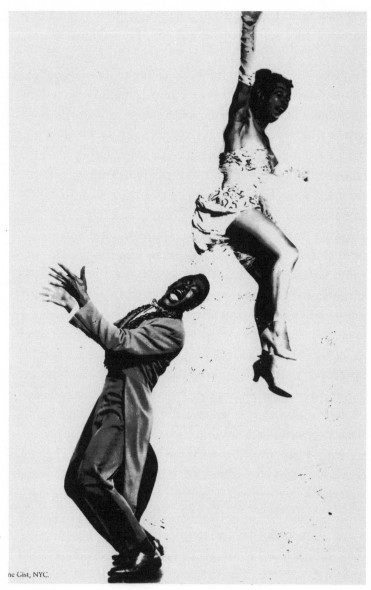

ne Gist, NYC.

Billy Ricker and Norma Miller dancing at
the Roxy Theater in 1952.

Harlem was hurting, and I could feel her pain. A meanness began to overtake her. Artistic black people were leaving, they were being replaced by disillusioned young people who wore their wickedness openly. Harlem began to look ugly to black citizens.

Among the hustlers dope began to replace the numbers, and the pushers were getting bold, pushing dope all over Harlem, and they didn't care who they were pushing it to. The addicts mostly preyed on older folks. Apartment break-ins, muggings, and all kinds of stealing became more common every day. One thing I want to stress is that the citizens of Harlem didn't bring in the dope. Dope was brought into Harlem by people with the resources to bring it into the country. Harlem was a convenient place to dump it, and a whole generation got wasted. No place was that more evident than in the music world. We lost many great musicians to dope. The saying in Harlem was, "Horse is boss." It controlled the mind and demanded everything from its users. The tragedy affected the entire community though, when the pushers needed new buyers, they started selling to young people and school children. First they sold in the high schools, then in the elementary schools. This had a huge negative impact on the community, and a lot of people found a way to leave. So did I.

Norma Miller Dancers

In 1952, while still in New York, I formed the Norma Miller Dancers. Billy Ricker, my former dance partner, joined this traveling dance revue. My own drummer, Mike Silva, traveled with us. We had the good fortune to inherit many of the former Lindy Hopper's jobs. Our first date was at the Apollo Theater. I didn't plan it but every time I had a new act, it debuted at the Apollo.

This was the beginning of the craze when vocal groups took the names of birds. It was the first time the Orioles starred in a show, and Mr. Schiffman put my act on the bill to add variety. My troupe included new, young dancers, following the pattern that Whitey had set when we started out.

The group included Frankie's son, Charles "Chazz" Young. When Frankie brought him on the scene, Chazz was seventeen years old, and because he had been raised by his mother, it was when I first learned that Frankie had a son. But after he danced for me, I had no doubts that he was Frankie Manning's. He danced just like his father, he showed that same natural grace and rhythm; the kid had it.

Our act continued at the Roxy Theater, where Sammy Rauch and Gae Foster became our managers. I was put in the Olsen and Johnson organization, and we became their opening act in *The Big Show* along with the Dancing

Waters. We did a jazz number and a big Cuban number, with the roller skaters on a big drum beating the tom-tom. There were twenty-four skaters, and it was the most exciting act in the show. We played the Chez Paris in Chicago, the Flamingo in Las Vegas, and The Mapes in Reno. But after that date Olsen and Johnson were in an accident while driving to Nebraska and the tour ended.

We next went to Australia with David Martin of the Tivoli Circuit touring the country from Melbourne to Perth in a show called *Coloured Rhapsody*. We toured Australia for nearly a year before another accident literally crashed down on us. In our sixth week of a new fifty-two week contract, my dancer Stoney Marteeni was caught in the fire curtain at the end of our big number. Someone had let the curtain down too soon, and as Stoney slid across the stage, the curtain hit him and broke his ankle. As I rushed to him I saw the twisted mess, raw bone with the white flesh dangling from it. It was all I could do to keep from passing out. I held his head and spoke to him until the ambulance came.

Stoney would recover, but it was going to be a long process. So, we regrouped and carried on until another dancer took sick. This time it was Billy Dotson, a divine dancer who had a special step called the "Butterfly." This step took a lot of wind out of him, and Billy was having a terrible time breathing and was constantly using an inhaler. Eventually we had to cut the step out altogether, but Billy became so ill he had to be hospitalized. Now we were down to two boys and four girls. I did everything I could think of to fill the gap, but it just didn't work. When we reached Sidney, the show was cancelled.

We managed to get Stoney and Billy back for the trip home and had to take a tramp steamer. It was a let down, but we had most of the ship to ourselves and relaxed for the entire twenty-four days it took to get back to the States. We went by way of Brisbane and Panama, and we finally ended up in Boston where we took a train back to New York and started rebuilding the act.

Then we joined the Count Basie show, becoming a part of the most exciting production on the road. It was an all-colored show, and it was swinging. The line up included George Kirby, Bill Bailey (brother of Pearl Bailey, and a great dancer), and the Herman Chitterson Trio. We went all the way back to the West Coast with this act. My kids in the show and I became good friends with the wonderful George Kirby. Things really heated up when we were booked in Las Vegas, the first all-black show to play the strip.

The show, including Basie, traveled by bus. But, Bill Bailey had just purchased his first Cadillac, and he decided to drive to Vegas by himself. We were booked into the Flamingo Hotel, but we were not allowed to stay on the strip because of our color—Las Vegas was as bad as Mississippi in those days. So we took up residence at Miss Shaw's Cabins on Van Buren. The bus would come to pick us up and take us to the strip at seven o'clock. The first night when the bus came, Bill Bailey had not arrived yet. We were worried; anything could happen to a black man driving cross country alone in those days. Especially driving a Cadillac. Hoping that he had driven directly to the Flamingo and would meet us there we got on the bus and headed for the strip. When we arrived at the hotel we got the word that Bill was in Las Vegas—New Mexico! When

he had come to a fork in the road he followed the sign for
Las Vegas, New Mexico instead of the one for Nevada.
Vegas was not yet popular with Easterners, and he just
guessed wrong. He missed the first night entirely.

We were doing two shows a night, eight o'clock and
midnight. When we were done we got our asses on the bus
and headed for the West side. We were not welcome in the
casinos. Between shows all we could do was stay in our
dressing rooms. Out of sheer boredom, George came up
with a great idea. We went around town on Fremont Street
and bought gambling paraphernalia. We got all the accesso-
ries for a craps game and spread the rag on some boxes
backstage. We got our own venture going, I cut the game,
and George handled the pit. We immediately captured
players back there; the band, the rest of the show, even the
hotel bosses came back and gave us a play. Although we
couldn't play at their tables, we didn't discriminate. They
were actually a nice bunch of guys, and they treated us very
well, it was just hotel policy.

Pearl Bailey was in town performing at Wilbur Clark's
Desert Inn. Because she was the star, she was welcomed at
the Desert Inn's tables. She came over to the Flamingo to
see our show, and on her way through the casino she took a
fling at the dice. They closed the table on her. It took a
moment before she realized what they were doing, but
when she did she was enraged.

"I don't have to spend my money where I'm not welcome, I can always play at the Desert Inn!"

We were backstage running a game while we waited for
the midnight show to hit. Pearl came back pissed, telling us
what had happened and ended up playing our tables.

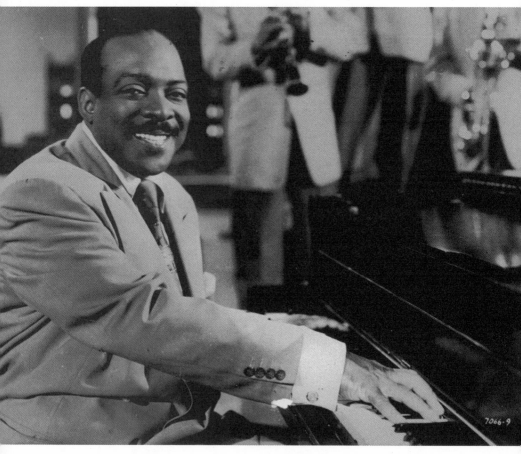

Count Basie.

Our tour ended in Las Vegas, but the band was going to L.A. to play a date at the Oasis nightclub, and we had a free ride on the bus. George and I had done very well with our craps game, and we decided to take a chance on picking up work there. So when the band got ready to leave for L.A. we packed up our dancers, and with high hopes and a suitcase full of silver dollars we headed for the West Coast.

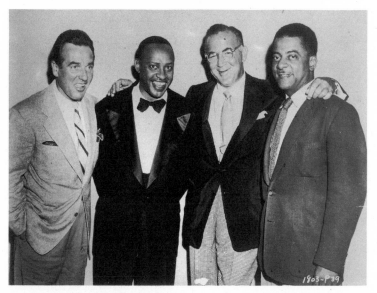

Gene Krupa, Lionel Hampton, Benny Goodman, and Teddy Wilson (left to right).

"You could say that the Count created swingin' jazz, Shaw intellectualized it, and the Duke did something entirely different—elegant and original. All Duke's men had the same independence; they were absolute pros, in the business for many years."

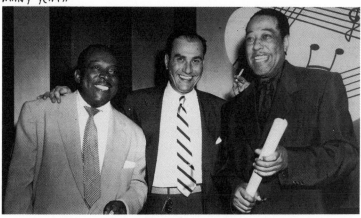

Count Basie, Artie Shaw, and Duke Ellington (left to right).

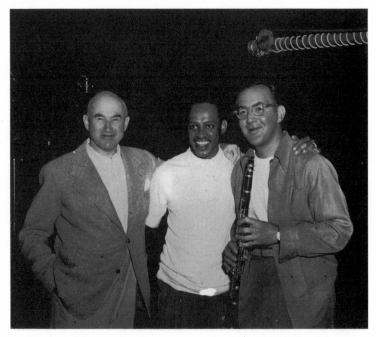

Samuel Goldwyn, Lionel Hampton, and Benny Goodman (left to right).

My dear friend Mrs. T and her lovely daughter Lena had a big house on Cimmaron (before the freeway), and they were able to put a few of my dancers up. Another friend, Johnny, accommodated those she couldn't, and George and I checked into the Watkins Hotel on Western and Adams.

George, being an incredible impressionist and marvelous at whatever he did had a plan to get a job with the Basie band on opening night at the Oasis. Basie used to bring the band on the stage one person at a time. He would go up and plunk at the piano, giving the cue. Then the drummer would enter and so on until the entire band was assembled. This night, without any planning or warning, George went on the stage instead of Basie, impersonating him. The audience loved it, and Basie just stood on the side and let it go, he, too, was entertained by George.

When that show was over and the band was backstage preparing for the next show, everyone was including George in the instructions. At this point he had not been hired by Basie, but the routine was such a hit with the audience that they agreed to hire him.

When this engagement ended, the Basie band headed up the coast and then back east. George and I stayed in Los Angeles. We put together a show and got some much needed dates at the Oasis. By that time any work was a big help. When you're supporting fourteen people, not even a suitcase full of silver dollars can last too long.

We had just landed some television work when I got a call from Basie's manager. He wanted George Kirby and my act to rejoin the Basie Band in Cleveland, Ohio.

"Do you think you can make it?" he asked.

"Shit yeah, we can make it!" I told him, not thinking about the fact we would have only three days to travel there after we finished the television shoot, and I had no idea what we would use for transportation.

When I told George what I'd agreed to, he asked me, "Do you think we can make it?"

I said, "We got to make it, we ain't got a choice."

Using the rest of our Vegas money and with a friend putting up the rest, we managed to hustle up two cars, a DeSoto station wagon and a Kaiser Frasier. I arranged to be paid right away for the television gig so we could leave directly from the studio.

So there began the great cross-country trek; Billy and four of the guys riding with me in the Kaiser Fraiser,

George, all six of the girls, and one of the guys in the station wagon.

If ever there was a perfect copilot to take an arduous trip across the country with, it was George Kirby. It was a rough excursion, but we laughed and sang all the way. When we started out the sun was shining, and we were in summer clothes. But we drove into winter—and into a snow storm. George appeared to be pulling off the road and waved. I followed him off the road, not realizing that he was stuck, until I was stuck too. There we were in the middle of nowhere, two cars full of dancers, stranded. Wrapped in blankets we retrieved from the trunk, the guys got out to push, but they slipped and slid on the ice, and we got nowhere. Cold as hell, we spent the entire night in that spot.

As the sun rose the next morning, we saw we were near a farm house. The folks there gave us coffee and pulled us out of the snow.

We were on a very tight schedule, and the only way we were going to make it was to keep the cars moving. But, George and I were the only ones with driver's licenses. We had no choice but to have the dancers take turns at the wheel while we slept. We went as fast as the cars would go. Nathan, the dancer riding with George, was taking a turn at the wheel, and I was following behind him when we were both pulled over. By the time the cop got to the window of the station wagon, the dancers had managed to get George into the driver's seat and had put the cap that Nathan was wearing onto George's head. Now, George was a very large man, and Nathan was a little guy, so the cap just sat on top of George's head and looked asinine.

We had to follow the policeman to a little courtroom off the side of the freeway where we were fined by the judge, "forty-five dollars, or forty-five days in jail." Meanwhile George, who was a very sound sleeper, still didn't know what in the hell was going on, or why he was being fined. He stood there, still half asleep with that ridiculous cap on his head, and I could only laugh.

"I'll pay the fine," I told the judge.

"For what?" George said.

I gave George a "Just shut up!" look. I paid the fine and dragged his ass out of there before he could ask any more questions. We made it to the theater in time for the first show.

After the date in Cleveland we returned to New York. We were stunned to see all of the changes that had taken place in the dance world. Frankie had abandoned his dance act and had gone to work for the post office. Someone called Momma Lou had entered the big space left by Whitey's death and Frankie's departure.

The *Daily News* was no longer sponsoring the Harvest Moon Ball, so Momma Lou started her own. For the next thirty years she trained dancers and kept dancing alive for black dancers; her shows were well known throughout the state. She had a style that was reminiscent of Whitey's Lindy Hoppers. Her dancers had speed and were able to capture the flying steps that were most essential to rhythm dancing. With her command of the theatrical style of dancing, she was able to replace Whitey's dancers. We appreciated her efforts, grateful that she took the challenge to help the dance survive.

Back on the road, the Norma Miller Dancers rejoined

Olsen and Johnson, playing mostly large arenas, this time with the Skating Vanities.

In 1956, Murray Weinger and Benny Davis put together the *Cotton Club Show* starring Cab Calloway, Sallie Blair, Lonnie Satin, George Kirby, and the Norma Miller Dancers. Mervyn Nelson was the producer and the show broke all racial barriers. We were to be the first all-black show to play the Beach Comber in Miami Beach.

During rehearsal racial tensions surfaced. Permits were needed to perform on the beach. The day of our big dress rehearsal there were headlines in the *Miami Sun* telling Murray Weinger that they didn't want his colored show on the beach. We were in our dressing rooms when pandemonium broke loose. We could hear voices in the alley behind the building and what sounded like pounding on the walls. I was terrified, I ran to the kitchen and hid beneath the butcher block, sure that I was about to be lynched. When the voices died down, I was surprised to hear George Kirby laughing, hysterically. Then I found out what had really happened—it was just George in the alley imitating a mob and throwing trash cans around trying to scare the hell out of us. He did. At the time I wanted to strangle George, but later we all had a great laugh.

The *Cotton Club Show* turned out to be a hit in Miami Beach, and it was there that I took my first stab at comedy. We did a skit based on *Romeo and Juliet* in which I played Juliet opposite Cab Calloway as my "Rock 'n' Roll Romeo." He entered carrying a guitar and wearing a short jacket, a large hat with colorful plumes, and bright yellow tights! I was up in the window of the castle looking down, and I nearly cracked up when I saw him. It was a great show.

We played Miami Beach for three consecutive years, returning the next year for the second edition of the *Cotton Club Show* with Cab Calloway and the Step Brothers, and the third time, in 1958, in *Jump for Joy* with Duke Ellington and Barbara McNair.

By 1960 ballroom dancing was becoming more free-lance. The Twist was taking the country by storm. Dancers began breaking away from each other and doing their own thing. Nothing resembled a partner dance anymore, it seemed everyone wanted to be on their own. It seemed to me that all style went out of ballroom dancing. Small combos were replacing the big bands, and the be-pop style of music was getting people to sit down and listen to the music, rather than dance to it.

I took so much of Whitey with me in my work. My basic dancing was still rooted in jazz, but now I had also added a jungle flavor to my numbers. For example, I choreographed Stan Kenton's "Cuban Episode" which had a Swing Latin beat.

Mike Silva, my drummer, traveled with me. I didn't use the congo drums as most dance groups did, Mike was a jazz drummer. Like my dancers, he was young. He played his first job in show business with me. His mentor was Joe Jones, Count Basie's drummer; he even looked like Joe. He added the Swing beat to my dance numbers, and just like the dancers, he rehearsed with us every day as part of the group. He became so proficient at following the dancers that everywhere we appeared, the stars would invariably ask me to let my drummer play for them. While we were at the Town Casino with Billy Daniels, he asked me to let Michael play for him. Of course I never objected, I felt the more experience Mike gained, the better he would be with us. At the time Sammy Davis, Jr., was a part of his uncle's act, the Will Masten Trio. Sammy saw Mike performing with us, at the time, and he told me he was impressed with him. So impressed, in fact, that the next time he saw Mike he asked him to join his own act.

He stole my drummer!

Mike had been with me for so long, it was hard to let him go. He was with us from the beginning of the Norma Miller Dancers. When we had appeared in the big arenas with the Skating Vanities, the company used Mike as the drummer for the show. He had been across Australia on the Tivoli Circuit with us, and over all those years he had developed into one of the finest percussionists I had ever heard. I really missed him when he left, after all the time we had spent working together as an act, it was like losing one of my own kids. But a break like playing for Sammy Davis, Jr., was nothing to pass up, and I was happy for Mike. Of course, that didn't keep me from wanting to kill Sammy.

JOE WILLIAMS was raised in Chicago. Blessed with a marvelous baritone voice, he began his career in the late '30s. He worked with a variety of jazz bands including those of Lionel Hampton, Coleman Hawkins, Andy Kirk, and Jimmie Noone, but attained his greatest notoriety from his work with Count Basie, performing such swingers as "Every Day I Have the Blues" and "All Right, Okay, You Win." The multifaceted Joe Williams now lives in Las Vegas where he frequently performs and, as he says, is "just havin' a good time."

When we came along, we were lucky enough to come along when the bands played for dancing in the dance halls, the Savoy Ballrooms in New York and Chicago. All over the country wherever you went there were dance halls, and the people went to them to dance. The bands played Swing music, and it felt so good that the dancers would dance from the first number to the very last note. Really, as a musician you did it as much for the dancing as you did for the music. All of that was together at one time, it was one great communication, and it never has been like that since.

I played the Savoy with Mr. Basie—I was with him from 1955 to 1961—we played dances all over the country. When the band would see real fine dancers, the musicians would try to become a part of what they were doing. Really, the dancers inspired the musicians and vice versa. If the musicians did something exceptional, it inspired the dancers to do something exceptional, and then the dancers would inspire the musicians to do even more. It was a party, it was the best.

Norma Miller was the mean lean instigator. She was the hottest dancer as a kid, you understand. She was impossible really. She was so great in fact, that she wound up being the choreographer. She was always the leader. She ended up being right out front. That was hard because she never felt she was that pretty to be out in front leading all the girls, but she danced so good, she made the other girls look clumsy. Norma could look like a plain Jane, until she got out there on the floor and the music hit her. Then she started dancing, and she was the most exciting thing you ever saw, and that's the truth.

—Joe Williams

On the Road Again

The Norma Miller Dancers enjoyed many successful years performing on the road with the greats of show business, but by the early 1960s it was no longer profitable to travel in so large a group. I was forced to trim down the act; I chose to release the girls and we became, Norma Miller and Her Jazzmen—Charles "Chazz" Young, Billy Dotson, Raymond Scott (who was later replaced by the wonderful Sterling), and, of course, my long time partner Billy Ricker.

My dancers were the best. Chazz (Frankie Manning's son) was with me from the time he was seventeen. He is a fantastic performer with true rhythm and grace, and he is still dancing today. He has always remained a dear friend. Billy Dotson was a superb dancer and a real party guy. He skated professionally with Maple Fairbanks before coming to dance with me, but there was very little work for professional skaters (especially black ones). He had a natural rhythm and he danced as if he were made of elastic. Raymond Scott was also a fine dancer, and he was the only dancer I ever had to fire. One time he came to rehearsal drunk, something that I found intolerable. My dancers could do whatever they wanted on their own time, but if it affected the act, it was over. Sterling replaced Raymond. He also was an exceptional dancer. He was another skater and a fine addition to the Jazzmen. And Billy Ricker, a partner of

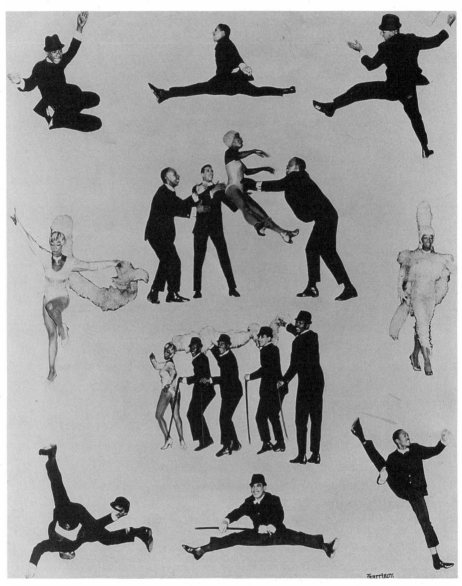

*Norma Miller and Her Jazzmen opened with Sammy Davis, Jr.,
at the Latin Casino in 1963.*

mine since our teen years, was a marvelous dancer and a great person. Billy was one of the best friends I ever had. I loved all of my dancers, and no matter what adversities we may have encountered, we always managed to have a great time together.

Our first date with the Jazzmen was a ten-month stay in London in the *Colored Express*. From there we went to Atlantic City, to the Club Harlem where we played the entire summer. Sammy Davis, Jr., came for the last two weeks. The engagement was huge. For two weeks Kentucky Street was so packed you couldn't walk on the street. Sammy was even awarded a plaque for bringing so much business to Atlantic City. We went on to perform with Sammy Davis, Jr., in Cherry Hill, at the Latin Casino.

In 1963 we joined the Count Basie show again. This time it was the greatest jazz show ever assembled. It was the Basie Band, with Joe Williams, Lambert, Hendricks and Ross, Redd Foxx, and the great Baby Lawrence. We played the Apollo Theater, the Howard in Washington, the Royal in Baltimore, and the Tivoli in Chicago.

It was in Chicago, when we were performing a Saturday matinée with Redd Foxx, that we heard that Martin Luther King, Jr., and his followers were being beaten by Eugene "Bull" Connor and his thugs in Birmingham, Alabama. Everyone in the show was upset. We all were keeping up with the news of the civil-rights movement, and I guess we all felt guilty about being on the sidelines and not out there with King. We tried to do something to help—we sent contributions and, later, blankets for the folks who marched on Washington and were living in those skimpy tents—but we were hundreds of miles away from where the really courageous people were making a stand. I guess the news made a lot of us feel like cowards. This was an all-black show for an all-black audience, so the same kinds of things must have been going through the audience's minds too.

We had to do a midnight show that Saturday, our last show at the theater. When my act came off stage, Redd was not in the wings waiting for us as he usually was. I hadn't seen him since the evening show and was told no one else had either. This was unusual, and I began to worry that something might be wrong. We were all still pretty shaken by the news from Birmingham, and we waited in the wings to see if Redd would step through the curtain to do his act as usual. We were relieved when he did, but were unprepared for what he did.

The house was packed, five thousand people were there. Redd stepped out on the stage, and the first thing he did was remove his hat and drop his head. His head was wrapped in a large gauze bandage, shaped like a cross, and it was red, like blood.

Redd lifted his head and his first words were, "Those folks ain't kiddin' down there."

The house roared with laughter, and it released the tensions backstage, we also roared. It was the mark of a great comedian to take a tragic moment and turn it into a laugh, only Redd could make a joke out of such turmoil and break a crowd up like that.

Our engagement was over, and the Basie Band was heading back to California, so I loaded up my Jazzmen and decided to ride back with them. I had a lot of friends in L.A. and felt confident we could pick up some work there. Nick Castle was kind enough to set up an audition for us.

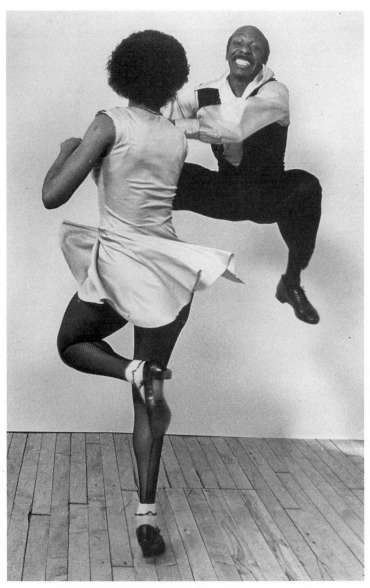

Debbie Williams and Chazz Young in 1984.

The audition was at Ciro's and the Basie Band offered to help me out. The audition started, and one at a time, as was their style, the Basie Band filed in and played for me. I thought it was the greatest, but the strategy backfired. The management said that anyone who could get Basie to play an audition for them didn't need a job!

So, I was stuck in California with four dancers and no job. We were staying at the Roosevelt Hotel, and I couldn't pay the bill. Nick Castle rescued me by paying it. I owed him that seven hundred and fifty dollars until he died.

Eventually we got a week's work with the Redd Foxx show at the Summit in Los Angeles. Betty Jean, Redd's wife at the time, was singing in the show too. After our last night we were preparing to leave town, and I went out with Redd and his wife. While we were driving in the car Betty Jean, who was gorgeous, but not a great singer, asked us, "How'd I sound tonight?"

Redd replied, "Honey, you hit a note tonight that curdled the drinks."

After this engagement, it was back across the globe; Australia, Hong Kong, Taiwan. Times became increasingly difficult, and the strain of being responsible for my group of dancers began to wear on me, so in 1968, when once again our funds were low, I decided it was time to disband the act.

I had an offer from Redd Foxx who thought I was a natural at comedy. He had told me that comedy would take me a lot further than dancing. That made sense to me, and I took his offer. My dancers returned to New York, and I went to Los Angeles where Redd had opened a club at La Cienega and Beverly. Redd began to teach me his craft, and I began my comedy career. He taught me timing and delivery, and before long I was earning my keep as a comedienne. I enjoyed the freedom of being responsible for only myself.

While in L.A. I got in touch with Roy Glenn. He had married a piano player in 1963, and they had a son, Larry. We had remained friends, and it was great to see him again. He was the one love of my life.

The Vietnam War was raging, and the country's unrest continued. Meanwhile I kept plugging away at comedy, under the wing of Redd Foxx. I began receiving offers to travel as a comedienne, and in the winter of 1971 I contracted to do a tour in Vietnam.

Christmas that year was especially happy, I was preparing for my tour and excited about my career in comedy. Roy dropped over for a holiday visit, and we spent the evening chatting about old times and, of course, our careers. His acting career was going very well, and I was happy for him. As he left that night, we embraced, and promised to stay in touch.

In February of 1972 I arrived in Vietnam. Troops had begun to pull out, and it appeared our presence there soon would end. Spirits were lifting, and we were glad to be there to raise them a little higher.

Every morning I would pick up a copy of the *Stars and Stripes* to stay in touch with the news from home. One morning, I wished I had not. We were performing in Da Nang and I grabbed the paper, as usual. I was shocked by the caption, "Actor Roy Glenn Succumbs to Heart Attack." I thought my own heart would stop. I read the article, then I reread it. It couldn't be true. I had just seen him a couple of months before. But there it was; my Roy was gone.

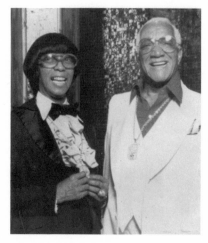

"my dear friend Redd and i were at caesar's palace in Las vegas on the night of the Larry Holmes— muhammad Ali fight in 1978."

Norma Miller and Redd Foxx.

Returning to the States wasn't possible, in fact I had a show to do that night and the show must always go on. There was no time to grieve, my schedule would not allow it. I finished my tour in Vietnam amazed at how cruel life could be.

Back in Los Angeles, I returned to the Redd Foxx Club. I was happy to be at home in the States, I loved being involved with Redd and with comedy. No matter how bad things got, people were always laughing. I started reading everything I could find on comedy, especially on black comics.

In 1974 I conceived the idea of a book. Redd and I collaborated, and we developed the *Redd Foxx Encyclopedia of Humor*. While doing the research and writing the book, I continued performing as a comic.

In 1977 I accompanied Redd to Las Vegas where I opened his show at the Hacienda Hotel. Soon after, our book was completed and published. I was thrilled. Redd

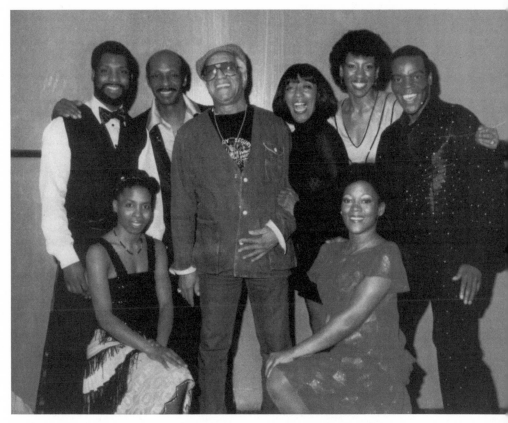

The New Jazz Dancers with Redd Foxx at the Playboy Club in Atlantic City in 1984. In rear are Clyde Wilder, Chazz Young, Redd Foxx, Norma Miller, Debbie Williams, and Stoney Martini; in front are Amaniyea Payne and Darlene Gist.

had approved the details of the project as they had come up, but had not wanted to be involved in the actual writing. Nonetheless I was sure that he, too, would be thrilled now that the project was completed.

One afternoon when I was at the mall, I visited Dalton's book store. There it was, the *Redd Foxx Encyclopedia of Humor* in front of the display window. I couldn't wait to tell Redd and ran to a pay telephone.

When he answered I told him how fabulous it was. I was at the mall, and our book was displayed, right in the front window! His reaction nearly knocked me over. He said it had to be taken down right away. I thought he'd lost his mind. Then he told me that he hated the cover—of which he had approved—and he wanted it off the shelves. He told me to take care of it and hung up! I stood there in shock. I couldn't believe what he had said. After all that work, how could he say such a thing?

Later I learned that one of Redd's friends, Slappy, had put the idea into his head that I was going to make a fortune from his name and that he wouldn't get his share of it. It ended sadly, and I was very disappointed.

I decided to stay on in Las Vegas. Things had changed a great deal since the early days when I had played there, and there were plenty of projects for me. One of my favorite productions was *Let Me Off Uptown* with Doris Troy, Bobby Wade, and Valerie Jackson.

In 1982 I returned to New York and Mama; healthy, sexless, still single, and broke.

"This show was based on *Ain't misbehavin'* and featured the works of black composers."

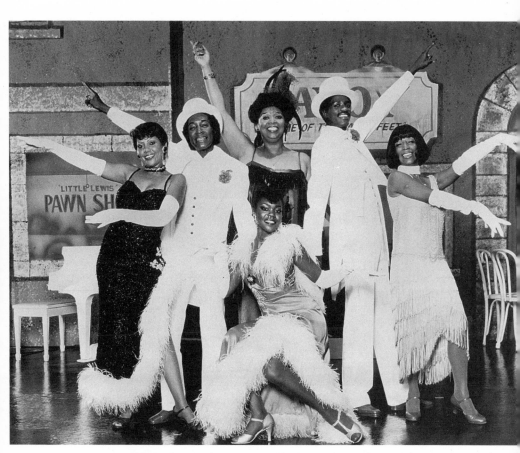

Auserita, Bobby Wade, Doris Troy, Ivory Wheeler, Norma Miller, and Valerie Jackson in Let Me off Uptown *at the Tropicana in 1981.*

Jon Hendricks was born in 1921 in Newark, Ohio. By the time he reached his teens, he and his family moved to Toledo where he began making regular radio appearances. It was there that he briefly met the amazing saxophonist Charlie Parker; the result was that Jon pursued music professionally. In 1958 he formed Lambert, Hendricks and Ross, a trio that mastered vocalese. After the trio dissolved in 1964, Jon developed Jon Hendricks and Company. Performing worldwide through the years, Mr. Hendricks has won many prestigious awards, including five Grammy awards for Manhattan Transfer's 1985 album *Vocalese*. His CBS television documentary, *Somewhere to Lay My Weary Head*, in which he starred and narrated, won Emmy, Iris, and Peabody awards. The versatile Jon Hendricks and Company currently perform a variety of programs, ranging from historical jazz performances to the contemporary. During his long career, Hendricks has performed with many of the greatest jazz musicians. His career is still in full swing, taking him on tour around the globe.

I never actually made it to the Savoy Ballroom, when I went to New York during the war I only had three days and there wasn't time. But I did know all the cats in all the bands that played there. I had been into music all my life. Swing was the way you danced in the '30s, the '40s, and even into the '50s, that was it.

Because of our love for Swing music, Dave Lambert and I decided to put something together. At the time we were living together; we had both been through a divorce and we didn't have any money, so I moved into his two bedroom flat.

There were great things happening in music at the time. There was Count Basie and his orchestra, Andy Kirk and his orchestra, McKinney's Cotton Pickers, and Frank Lightfoot and his orchestra. All the sections of the

country had their orchestras. There was a cat out of
Detroit named King Kovaks who had a great orchestra
with a lot of cats in it from Chicago. All these people
played the music that the dancers at the Savoy danced to.
It was the music. It was the only kind of music that really
was in show business. Even stage shows in the theaters
had jazz bands. Everything fit that music, and we all
loved it. Dave and I were trying to figure a way to use the
music we loved, and make a living out of it.

So we said, "What can we do?"

Dave said "What about Count Basie?"

And I said, "Yeah, I like Basie too."

So, we wrote the album idea for Sing A Song With
Basie, then we had to sell it to a record company, and that
took us about eight months. Dave had conducted vocal
groups behind a lot of the popular stars of the day. He did
"Hawaiian War Chant" for Jo Stafford. All the time he
called the group the Dave Lambert Singers. I had done a
couple of these gigs with Dave and this group to make
some money.

When we did the thing with Basie we had Sonny
Payne, Eddie Jones, Freddy Green, and a cat name Nat
Pierce who sounded just like Basie, in the line up.

We went in the studio with the Dave Lambert
Singers, there were twelve of them. So, we got in the
studio with them and realized they couldn't Swing. Well,
we had to make some changes, because you can't sing to
Count Basie or dance to Count Basie if you don't know
how to Swing. You can't even come near Count Basie if
you can't Swing. You might as well stay in bed, don't
even get up! Cause that is what that band is, was, and
always will be about.

There was one girl there, Annie Ross, who had come

over to New York from London in a show called Cranks.
The young Anthony Newly also made his debut in that
show. He and Annie were starving at the time, they were
doing nothing but this show on Broadway which wasn't
making that much money. They were both very good
people, so, we listened to Annie. We had heard her on
the Prestige records that she had done, Farmers Market
and Twistin', so we knew that she was hip. So we went
to the guy who had produced those records. We had
already lost twelve hundred and fifty dollars with those
other singers, and that was a lot of money in those days,
it was a fortune, and we were facing complete disaster.

The producer asked "What can we do?"

So Dave told him, "We'll have to multitrack."

We both asked Dave "What's multitrack?"

Nobody knew what that was. Dave explained we
would have to record all three of us together, Dave,
Annie, and me on one tape and get the three voices
together and then take that tape off and run a new one
with three voices more and so on until we had the
harmonies we were looking for. That was the first time
that had ever been done in the history of the music
business.

The words were important to me. I thought they were
very extraordinary, not because they were mine, I just
thought that the people would be able to follow along with
the songs if they could see the words. So we printed the
words on the back of the album.

People take those two things for granted now because
everybody does it, but we were the first. On top of that,
what we were doing on the album became known as a new
musical art form, vocalese, we invented that. That album,
Sing a Song with Basie is now in its umpteenth reissue on

GIP *and has been steadily selling at all times, somewhere in the world, ever since it was first released in 1958. It won the first jazz Grammy award.*

We live in a country that has the most vibrant cultural art form in history. We did it, Swing music is ours. It is a great legacy for our children, but we are being rapidly deculturized on a national level. There are a lot of young Negro people being deculturized in America. I use the word "Negro" advisedly; a word I would use as an alternative would be Afro-American because when you use the term black, then you put yourself with every other black person on the earth, and the only dark skinned people who produced this culture are us. Not all the blacks in Africa produced this, we're the ones, and we are American Negro people or Afro-Americans or niggers. As my dear friend Redd Foxx said, "You got to watch these black people, they're holding us niggers back!"

There is a lot of talk about all the "advancements" going on in music. You mean to tell me what's going on when you turn on your radio is an advancement? Someone must be just plain lying to tell me that over Louis Armstrong, Duke Ellington, Count Basie, Miles, and Dizzy that this crap that is going on today is an advancement. This is no advancement, this is a regression. This is a step way back. There is a regression of a serious nature here. That's what I hope this book reminds people. People need to see what they've turned away from and what they're turning toward. I can see if you turn away from one thing and you turn to something much more beautiful. But if you turn away from the most beautiful thing on the planet, to something that's flat out ridiculous, then something is wrong, and you're in serious trouble. Swing is the most beautiful thing I have ever discovered. I

*am seventy-two now, and I wouldn't stop doin' what I'm
doin' for nothing you can say on this earth. There's
nothing you can say on this planet that would stop me
from doing what I've been doing all my life, because it's
that beautiful. You want to know how beautiful it is?
That's how beautiful it is.*

—Jon Hendricks

Swingin' into the Future

I had been away from New York a long time, and naturally the first place I visited was Harlem. As I walked through the streets of Harlem, I was flooded with memories. It was all changed now. It brought tears to my eyes, seeing what was left of that great time in history. So much musical history had occurred there. It was the home of the big bands—Chick Webb, the Savoy Sultans, Benny Goodman, Teddy Hill, Willie Bryant, Count Basie—they had all played there. Ella Fitzgerald and Billie Holiday had begun their careers there. But there was no sign of them now. The Swing music and Swing dance that once thrived there should have been preserved, like New Orleans jazz. Jazz came from New Orleans, and Swing came from Harlem—from the Savoy Ballroom.

There should be a plaque at the site of the Savoy Ballroom to let future generations know that this is where the great bands had played and the dance was created. Standing where the Savoy had been, recalling the memories of the world that I had once lived in, I felt inspired to record the events that had taken place there.

When I told Mama what I wanted to do she looked at me as though I were crazy.

"You got no money, no job, and you want to write a book? You got to be out of your mind!"

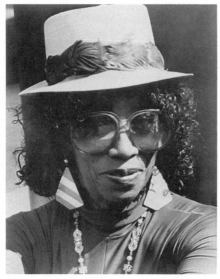

Norma Miller, 1984.

"Here I am wearing my mentor Buck Clayton's hat."

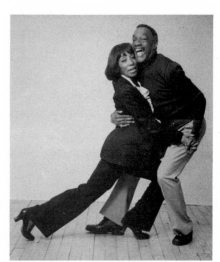

*Norma Miller and
Billy Ricker dancing at
the Village Gate,
New York, 1984.*

Still, I knew the story had to be told. And I also knew
that Mama was right—I had to find work—but I wasn't
going to forget about the book. It was on my mind all the
time as I got back into the swing of things and looked up a
number of my old dancing associates. One was Al Minns.
He was teaching Lindy dancing at the Sandra Cameron
Dance Center on West 20th Street. His pupils, mostly young
white kids who loved the Lindy, were always asking him to
bring them uptown, and finally he did. They enjoyed
themselves so much that it became a regular thing for them
to go uptown on Monday nights. It was great to see a
bunch of kids swinging in the old Harlem tradition.

I had told Al that I was planning a book, and one day he
called asking me to meet him at the Sandra Cameron Dance
Center, he wanted to introduce me to his manager at the
time, Larry Schultz, to talk about the book project. Larry
immediately started testing my knowledge of the Lindy
Hop. He seemed like a fairly nice guy, so I answered his
questions. At one point he put on a Swing record and asked
me to dance with him.

We had a couple of swings and he was surprised when I
said to him, "Al taught you to Swing."

"How did you know that?" he asked.

"Your Swing, with the leg gaping out at the side, it's
typical Al," I answered.

It wasn't long before he knew he was dealing with a
veteran of the dance. While we talked I told him of my
plans. We discussed how Al and I had been part of the
greatest Lindy Hop team in history. Talking about the old
gang, I discovered that he didn't know who Frank Manning
was.

"How is it that you don't know the greatest Lindy Hop dancer of all time when he is right here in New York City working at the post office? Well mister, if you don't know Frank Manning, you don't know nothing about Lindy."

Larry was eager to meet the other Lindy dancers who were still around, so we decided to get the whole gang back together. He wanted to meet Frankie right away, and I promised that the next time we met, Frankie would be there too.

Introducing Frankie to Larry Schultz proved to have a major effect on the teaching of the Lindy at the studio. Larry had brought someone with him to the meeting—a chubby, cute feller with an engaging smile who had a lot of equipment with him. He set up his screen and projector, and then we were introduced; enter Ernie Smith. He had the most extensive collection of films on black dancing I had ever imagined, many on the Lindy. I couldn't believe it, when he began the showing I let out a scream. He had my whole life in the Lindy on film! *A Day at the Races*, *Hellzapoppin'*. It was unbelievable. It was a wonderful

"when Stoney came back to the states after living in Iran for some years, he had a terrible illness. He was the first of my dancers to die of AIDS—we didn't even know what to call it then."

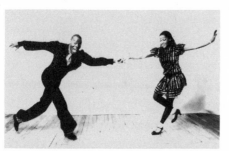

Stoney Martini and Darlene Gist.

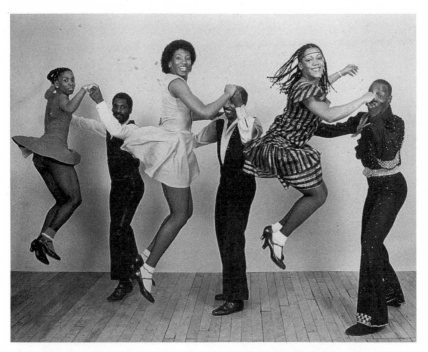

New Jazz Dancers Amaniyea Payne and Clyde Wilder, Debbie Williams and Chazz Young, and Darlene Gist and Stoney Martini (left to right).

moment for Frankie and me. It was the first time we had seen the films together, and thanks to Ernie Smith's love of the dance, they were preserved. We discussed Marshall Stearns' book *Jazz Dance* and the fact that in his chapter on the Savoy and the Lindy he had overlooked the fact that I was Leon James's partner at the time. He also didn't mention that Frankie Manning and I were in *Hellzapoppin'*. Thanks to Ernie Smith those films are around today, and the record can be set straight.

As the conversation went on we learned that Ernie was originally from Pittsburgh, and it was there that he had

"Billy, my long-time partner, and I were so close and had such a good working relationship that we never had an argument."

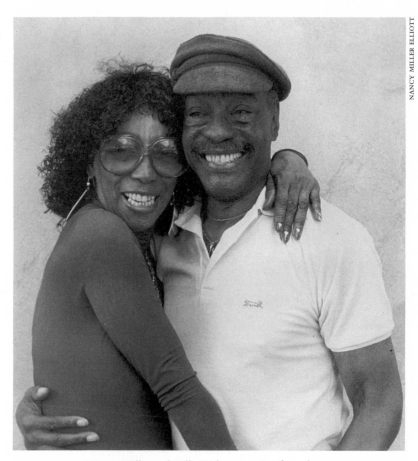

Norma Miller and Billy Ricker preparing for a show at the Village Gate in New York in 1984.

begun to dance the Lindy. He obviously had a real feeling for the contribution of black dancers to the world of Swing.

It was this meeting that lead to my choreographing a show that Larry Schultz produced at the Village Gate in 1984. It was the first time I had formed a new Lindy Hop group. It included my old friend Chazz Young, his dancing partner Debbie Williams, Clyde Wilder, and Amaniyea Payne. These were the dancers who began the new version of Swing dancing. I brought in the Jon Hendricks group, renowned for vocalese, a style of adding words to classic jazz instrumentals that Jon Hendricks created for the Lambert, Hendricks, and Ross trio. It was music that swings in the Basie manner.

The show was a decided success. Frankie Manning and Billy Ricker were in the opening night audience, and it gave me the opportunity to get together with my former partners. It was a great reunion, and it was lucky that it happened when it did. Shortly after, Al Minns became ill. We didn't know how serious it was at the time, but his condition steadily worsened. We lost a dear friend, and the dancers lost a fine teacher.

During the '80s Swing was regaining popularity. In London the craze inspired groups like the Jiving Lindy Hoppers and in Sweden, the Swedish Hot Shots. In this country a distinctly West Coast style developed with the West Coast Swing and Western Swing groups. In North Carolina they were doing the North Carolina Shag. They were even swinging on Beale Street. New York and Washington had their own Swing dance societies. In New York the C. and J. Band was formed to play the big-band style of music. When they opened at Small's Paradise in Harlem they got a terrific

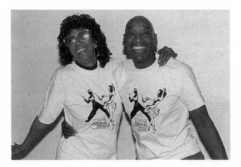

Norma Miller and Frankie Manning at a Cat
Club rehearsal in 1986.

response which started people dancing again at Small's
Paradise. Every Monday night it became a popular hangout
for Swingers. It became so popular that people began to
bring back the Lindy in the true Harlem tradition.

Monday night was the night for dancing, and even in
Al's absence the white kids kept coming from downtown to
dance. They were protected while they were there, Harlem
made sure nothing happened to them. With Al gone
though, the dancers needed a new teacher and I looked to
Frankie. Who better to teach dancers our style of dancing?
Who better to teach the new kids what it was all about?

In 1986 Frankie began a new career, this time as a
teacher. He was now well into his '70s, but despite all those
years spent working at the post office, he had never stopped
dancing and was in great shape. He was always an excellent
dancer, and his knowledge of Swing dancing was invaluable
to the young dancers. He started with Erin Stenens and her
partner Steve Mitchell. Now Steve teaches the style called
the Savoy Swing, he is one of the best stylists of Savoy
around today.

Frankie began working with a new group called the New

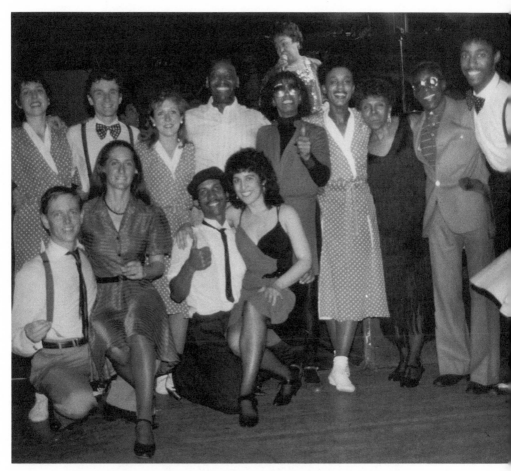

Frankie Manning and Norma Miller (center) *with Lindy Hoppers*
from England, California, and New York at
the Cat Club in New York City in 1986.

York Swing Dance Society (NYSDS). Within the NYSDS is a group of performers called the Big Apple Dancers—in memory of Whitey's Big Apple Dancers. Frankie taught them the original Big Apple that Whitey produced, and this became their signature. He also began teaching at the Sandra Cameron Dance Center and then took his style across the seas. He now teaches dance around the world. In Sweden he works with the Swedish Hot Shots, who worked with Al Minns before his death. They are the best professional Swing dancers in Sweden. Frankie also works with the Jiving Lindy Hoppers in London, who originally learned the American Lindy style from Pepsi Bethel. After their visit to the States, they worked with Frankie. They have developed into a fine theatrical group and are the top Swing dancers in England today.

Frankie teaches the Savoy style, and it's done the way the dance was created. It's what Lindy is all about. I believe he is the best dance instructor in New York today, he is the master teacher of Swing dancing, and people come from everywhere to take his classes.

One of Frankie's finest accomplishments was his choreography of the Broadway production of *Black and Blue* for which he won the prestigious Tony award, along with Henry LeTang, Fayard Nicholas, and Charles Atkins.

While I was still in New York, I had the opportunity to work with Alvin Ailey. One evening in '88 or '89 Ernie Smith and I were on our way to hear the pianist Jay McShann at Carnegie Hall, and we had the good fortune of running into Alvin on 57th Street on his way to the same performance. I hadn't seen Alvin for many years. The last time had been when we were appearing on the same bill in

Los Angeles at the old Earl Carroll Theater. At that time he
was a member of the Lester Horton Dancers along with
Jimmy Truitt. Carmen Delavellade was the star of that
group. Now Alvin had his own company, and they had
become world famous.

When he approached us there on 57th Street, he said,
"Norma, I've been trying to get in touch with you!"

"Well, I'm here, what's happening?" I asked. It was
always good to see him and he was looking fabulous. His
success was obvious.

He told me that he was planning a new ballet around Jay
McShann that would include jazz, and he wanted me to
work with him. I was a little skeptical, but I didn't say so. I
had never thought much of ballet dancers doing Swing.
They usually don't get the feel of it right, and I tell them,
"You Swing like my grandmother!" But years before, when
Alvin told me he wanted to form a great company of black
modern dancers, I didn't think it was possible. I knew the
talent was there, but I didn't think he could pull together all
the support he'd need. He proved me wrong on that; his
company was fabulously successful. So I heard him out. The
project sounded really exciting, and I told him I would love
to do it. Having my work with a great company like Alvin's
would give my Lindy Hop a more secure place in history.

Alvin and I got together the next day. I was very excited
about the project, and I planned to involve my long-time
partner Billy Ricker. But the project was just beginning to
take shape when Billy took sick. We lost him very quickly.
It was at Billy's wake that I announced that Frankie Manning and I would be working with the Alvin Ailey Company choreographing a new ballet.

For Frankie and me, working as choreographers together with the Alvin Ailey Company was one of the most rewarding moments in our dancing careers. The ballet "Opus McShann," made its debut at the Center Theater in December of 1990. Alvin invited Frankie and me to be part of the gala. George Falson directed the show, Bill Cosby emceed, Camille Cosby was the honored guest, and all of his dancers, past and present, were a part of the evening. This was the last time I would see Alvin alive. He was a fine artist and is greatly missed. I am proud to have "Opus McShann" a part of the repertoire of the Alvin Ailey Company.

Frankie and I were also involved in Spike Lee's production of *Malcolm X*. Otis Salid choreographed, but as his knowledge of Swing dancing was very limited, he brought in Frankie Manning to assist, and, I assisted Frankie. We appeared in a ballroom scene together. But I didn't think the results were authentic. Salid looked to the 1941 Universal picture *Hellzapoppin'* for his choreography of the dance number. His whole number worked around a series of air steps, but you could not distinguish one dancer from another. He also re-created this same choreography in *Swing Kids*, which was filmed in Czechoslovakia and set in Hitler's Germany (1938–1940). He used the same air steps on a ballroom floor, but he evidently didn't do his homework. Ballrooms had dance codes in 1938, and you never saw anyone thrown in the air in a ballroom unless it was in a contest. Swing dancing in a ballroom during that period was all floor work.

I was much happier with the results in Debbie Allen's made-for-television movie, *Stompin' at the Savoy*. She called and asked me to work with her on the project, and it was a pleasure to work with her. Debbie got right in and learned all of the steps with the dancers. She is a great dancer herself and understood what was involved. And the four featured actresses—Vanessa Williams, Lynn Whitfield, Jasmine Guy, and Vanessa Bell Calloway—also learned their routines and got with it. It is always a pleasure to work with pros, and these broads were real pros. Working with them was a gas! I guess I wasn't the only one who thought we had done a great job; I was nominated for an Emmy for best choreography.

By 1990 I was living in Las Vegas. I still traveled to wherever the good jobs were, but there was always so much happening in Vegas that I could stay busy right here. When the Debbie Reynolds Hotel and Casino opened there in June of 1993, one of the main attractions was a late night event they called Jazz and Eggs, which was held in the café. This featured the Ernie George Trio and included Jimmy Caesar as the emcee. These nights gave a variety of actors and singers the opportunity to get together and have some fun doing what they like to do best—entertain. Jimmy invited me to come by and I did. It turned out to be the regular hangout every weekend. The trio was great, and getting up and improvising gave me the opportunity to try out different bits without any pressure. One weekend I threw in a Lindy bit that I had done with Cisco Drayton, one of the dancers in *Malcolm X* and *Stompin' at the Savoy*. It was a spur of the moment thing that I ended my bit doing the Lindy Hop. I called it the Beat, and I did it to "Don't Mean a Thing, if it Ain't Got That Swing"—go figure. It was so successful that after that every time I got up to perform, they asked me to do the Beat.

"Jonathan is one of the great west coast—swing dancers. The west coast has a distinctive style, but we found lots of common ground in this show."

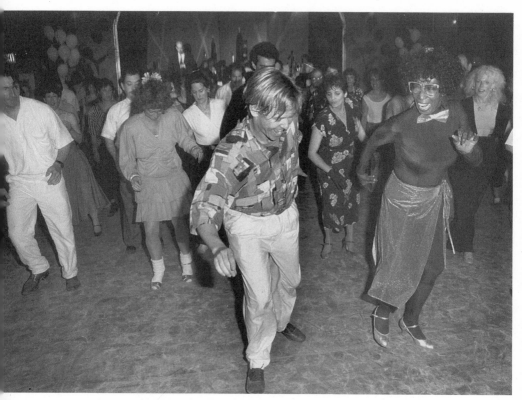

Jonathan Bixby and Norma Miller in the 1990 Boogie in the Berkshires.

One night I was up there doing my thing, and John Boffa, a movie director, happened to be in the house. He approached me and told me, "I want to put you in my movie."

Being an old hand at hearing bullshit, I replied, "Yeah, yeah . . ."

"I'm serious," he said, "who represents you?"

"See that white haired guy over there that looks like Buffalo Bill? Talk to him."

This was Harry Seybold, a talented producer and dear friend who frequently handled bookings for me in Las Vegas. In fact, Harry is the person who introduced me to Evette Jensen while she was working as his assistant producer. Well, Boffa was directing a movie in Florida called *Captiva* with Ernest Borgnine, Artie Johnson, and Bill Cobbs. I accepted a part in the movie, and we shot it in May of '94 in Fort Meyers, Florida. It was the first time I had appeared in film without dancing.

When I left Florida I went straight to New York, where the New York Swing Dance Society had planned a celebration for Frankie Manning's eightieth birthday over the Memorial day weekend. The affair was in appreciation for his dedication to helping them to preserve the dance. Dancers from all over the world came to honor Frankie, and it turned out to be the greatest reunion ever held for a dancer. The weekend was called Can't Top the Lindy Hop, and the events were held at the Roosevelt Hotel in Manhattan. There were workshops and panel discussions, and the weekend ended with an incredible birthday celebration. We danced all night long. Frankie was beaming. The world seemed right again, and I know Whitey would have been proud. It was the most fantastic gala in the history of Swing dance, and it was well earned.

So Swing dancing is still alive and well today, but like everything that's been around for more than fifty years, it has seen many changes. Basically, Swing dancing is dancing to the eight-bar beat of big band Swing music. The music inspired the dancers to innovate, and the dancers inspired the musicians.

The Lindy Hop started in Harlem with black dancers; when white bands became part of the Swing Era, white kids tended to follow bands like Benny Goodman's. It was about this time that the dance got faster and wilder. When the King of Swing, as they called Goodman, played the Paramount Theater in New York in 1938, the audience went wild and danced in the aisles. Goodman supposedly said that they looked like a bunch of Jitterbugs, and the name stuck. The promoters picked up the term and started hyping the new dance, the Jitterbug. To the rest of us, it looked like the Lindy Hop.

Although Harlem created it, the Lindy belongs to everyone. From the beginning there were dancers who were essentially performers and dancers who were social dancers. The social dancers would try to imitate the performers, and stage steps would show up on the ballroom floor. Whenever you would see someone trying aerial steps on a ballroom floor, you knew that they were copying something they had seen professionals do. Professional dancers felt that aerial steps were inappropriate—and downright dangerous—on a ballroom floor crowded with social dancers.

Whitey had developed a dance troupe to appear on the

professional stage, and the professional side was predominantly black. That was partly because Whitey was so committed to making his dancers the elite of Lindy Hop but also because the good white dancers were not encouraged to become professional. We saw any number of really good white dancers at the ballroom, but their families made them continue their educations. Kids who became entertainers would have been a disappointment. Harry Goldberg and his partner Ruthie were one of the best dance teams at the Savoy. Harry became a dentist. Jimmy Valentine was a Lindy Hopper even though he had only one leg; he did go into show business and became a partner of Peg Leg Bates. I met up with him in Las Vegas, where he lives with his wife; he still dances.

Black and white, professional and social dancers took Swing to all parts of the world. The dance picked up new techniques and regional styles, and all this give-and-take shaped the varieties of Swing that we have today.

It's all Lindy, and I hope the dancers continue to experiment and keep the interest alive. The dance is American, it was created in the Savoy Ballroom to the sounds of the big bands.

Looking back, it's been a wonderful time. Starting with the Harvest Moon Ball–champions going to Europe—Leon and Edith, Billy Hill and me. My first trip to England. The Ethel Waters group, Snookie and Willamae, George and Ella, my sister Dot and Johnny, Leon and me. The Australian group headed by Frankie, The Hot Mikado group, the making of *Hellzapoppin'* which led to a friendship with Nick Castle that lasted all through my dancing career. To the Norma Miller Dancers, to the Jazzmen, and later the

Norma Miller Jazz Dancers, playing the Playboy Club with Redd Foxx. . . . A lot of my dancers are gone today, but they will always hold a special place in my heart.

I've heard some of the dancers in workshops, discussing their concern for the future of Swing dance, but take it from me—you don't have to worry about Swing. It has gained its place alongside all great music. With composers like Duke Ellington, Count Basie, Chick Webb, Benny Goodman; Swing will always be with us. And, as long as there is Swing music, there will be Swing dancing.

"you can see the legendary jazz trumpeter Buck Clayton and his manager behind us."

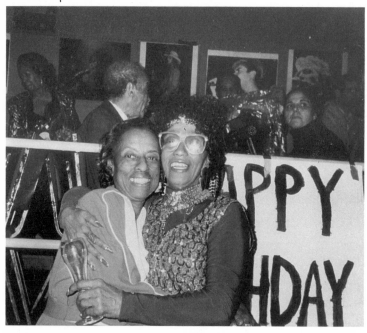

Dot and Norma at Norma's seventieth birthday party at the Cat Club.

Saying Goodbye

In October 1988 we lost my Mama. Over the years she had
lost interest in life, her zest seemed to have left her along
with her many friends who passed before her. It wasn't that
she was sick with any particular illness, but after eighty-
eight years, Mama had just grown tired. She was staying in
bed more often, and it worried us. She began to ramble on
about her mother, and she seemed to regret that she had
never returned to Barbados.

I was still living in New York, and my sister Dot and I
visited Mama everyday. We had always remained a very
close. Dot had taken Mama to the hospital a number of
times, and this annoyed Mama to no end. She insisted she
was fine. But Dot had worked at the Harlem Hospital for
twenty-seven years as a nurses' aide in the children's ward
and emergency room, so she knew more than a little about
illness.

Eventually we did have to put Mama in the hospital. It
was sad to see Mama losing interest in everything. She
always had been such a vibrant woman, full of energy and
pizazz. She had worked all her life, and it was as if she were
thoroughly tired of being retired.

During this time I was working with a small version of
the Savoy show that I had put together for Art Connection.
One weekend I had to go to Boston to appear at Brandeis

University. As usual I saw my mother before I left. It never
occurred to me that she might not be there when I returned. When I got back that Monday I telephoned Dot
who told me that Mama had passed during the night.

The realization that Mama was gone did not come easily.
For the first time in my life, nearly seventy years, she was
not there. With all of the loved ones I had lost through the
years, no loss could compare to this. When I got off the
phone I sat thinking about Mama, and her words came back
to me, "I'll suck salt before I ever leave my children in any
orphanage, I'll never separate them from me, ever!" She had
kept her word.

When we were children, she and her two sisters made a
home for all of us. Whoever had a job supported us, and
whoever was at home took care of the children. Mama's big
lesson was always that you had to figure out how to survive.
It was her strength and her spirit that carried me through
life. In difficult times it was her even keel that kept me
afloat. She always said to me, "If you don't like your
situation, you can always come home." It had made such a
difference in my life. I had grown up independent and had
taken on life fully. Never in my life did I have to compro-
mise what I really wanted, for a man or anyone else, because I knew my Mama would always be there for me.

I always say in my act, "Mother raised me in the twenti-
eth century, but she held on to mid-Victorian values." I
think she was resigned to her daughter being an old maid.
But it was different for me than it had been in her time. I
wasn't afraid of being a spinster as women were in my
mother's day. Actually, it gave me a special kind of freedom. When Whitey had asked me to take over the dancers

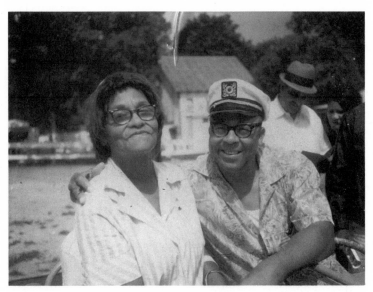

Alma Barker Miller and Peg Leg Bates at his resort.

for him, I was able to decline. I wanted my own dancers,
and I wanted my own company, and I set about getting
them—the Norma Miller Dancers. When I wanted to
change careers and become a comedienne, I did, and it was
my mother's indomitable spirit that led me all the way.

Dot did a fantastic job planning Mama's burial. She
arranged everything. All the dancers from the Swing Dance
Society attended the funeral. Plenty of people and laughter,
the kind of wake she would have enjoyed. She was dressed
beautifully, all in pink—her favorite color—and her makeup
was flawless. I bought her a mixed grey wig that was cute as
a button. As I looked at her in the coffin, I said to her,
"Mama, you're sharp kid." She would have been proud.

Whenever pressures got too heavy, and I felt like giving

253

up, her words always came back to me. And as we were driving to the cemetery, I remembered what she had told me, and her own mother had told her, "When you ain't got a horse, ride a cow."

My Mama was an inspiration. Because of her I was able to face adversity, and I dedicate the following to her:

It was a black woman who gave life to me
It was a black woman who said I'd be born free
To live my life full and with dignity
These are the things a black woman gave to me.

It was a black woman who carried the seed
Across the vast ocean, so that I'd be born free
She gave her love and truth to me
These are the things a black woman gave to me.

She said, "As you sow, so shall you reap
By the sweat of your brow, you'll earn your keep"
That black was a heavy load to bear
But God put no more on man, than he's able to bear.

It was a black woman who gave pride to me
And taught me that black was beautiful to be
She said to me, "Love and honor me"

These are the things a black woman gave to me.

Thanks Ma. I love you.

THE FUTURE OF THE LINDY
AND THE NEW YORK SWING DANCE SOCIETY

AN EPILOGUE
BY ROBERT P. CREASE

Popular dances occasionally have a powerful cultural and so-cial impact on the music of an era and on the way they foster contact between people across social, economic, and ethnic boundaries.

The Lindy was one of these dances. In the 1930s, big bands made their living by playing to Lindy Hoppers rather than through recording contracts or concerts. Half a century later, though on a different scale, the Lindy still carries surprising power, as is illustrated by the story of the New York Swing Dance Society.

Surely none of those who founded the organization had any idea where the dance would lead. I know I didn't. My road to acquaintanceship with the dance began with a class in the Jitterbug, which I took as a lark in 1982. It was the first dance class I'd ever taken, and I found it interesting—inter-esting enough so that I began to hang out with a few other Jitterbug enthusiasts at a Greenwich Village bar where they played music you could Jitterbug to on Thursday nights.

"Music you could Jitterbug to"—although it seems as strange to say now as it is embarrassing to admit, that was about the level of my musical sophistication at the time. I didn't know what Swing music was, nor did I have anything but the vaguest notion of the musical differences between Swing and Dixieland; or Swing, Rhythm 'n' Blues, and early Rock and Roll. All I knew and cared about was that I could do the triple-step, triple-step, back-step to certain music.

Then I met Al Minns. Al had been a member of Whitey's Lindy Hoppers, was one of Norma Miller's partners, and was a winner of the Harvest Moon Ball. All this meant nothing to me or any of the others in his class at the time; but he would teach us. Then all we knew was that he was an old-timer who was offering Lindy Hop lessons at the Sandra Cameron Dance Center, and he could help us to improve our dancing.

But thanks to Al we soon discovered entirely new dimensions of the dance, of the music, and of history. It's not that he was a good teacher; he wasn't. He could not explain steps very well, often miscounted the timing, constantly mixed up the men's and women's steps (he did both naturally, thanks to his years giving exhibitions for Marshall Stearns, in which he danced with Leon James), and was periodically late or even absent from class. Al was inspirational rather than instructional. He would throw himself into a swing-out, or into his signature rubberlegs step, or just improvise, and suddenly we could see what dancing was all about. We could see that it had nothing to do with repeating patterns correctly, but with throwing your body into the music.

After class we would retire to a nearby bar and Al would tell us stories of Harlem during the '30s—of nightclubs like Small's Paradise and Connie's Inn, of ballrooms like the Savoy and the Renaissance, and of dancers like Shorty Snowden, Rabbit, Twist Mouth George, Frankie Manning, and Norma Miller. He'd tell us of winning the Harvest Moon Ball in 1938; of filming *Hellzapoppin'*; of his trip to Brazil, and how Norma charmed Orson Wells; of struggling to keep the Lindy alive through exhibitions for Marshall Stearns in the 1950s and the 1960s; of being introduced by Langston Hughes at the Newport Jazz Festival; and of how the exhibitions came to an end in 1966 with Stearns's death.

Thanks to Minns's classes, our music listening habits changed. We grew to appreciate the music more, and learned that we had to listen to it carefully in order to dance to it. We quickly learned to loathe Glenn Miller's version of "In the Mood," and to appreciate the fact that it almost didn't Swing. I remember receiving an hour-long lecture from Al when I inadvertently put on a Dixieland record at a dance and said it would make good Swing dancing music. We learned to pick out the Basie beat from the Ellington sound, to appreciate bands like Lucky Millinder and Jimmie Lunceford, and even to recognize some of the musicians.

Our involvement with the dance moved us into yet another dimension in February 1984, when, from jazz disc jockey Phil Schaap, we learned that the newly reopened Small's Paradise was offering dancing to big band music on Monday nights. I still remember the first time I walked into the club, on Adam Clayton Powell, Jr. Boulevard at 135th Street, with a few friends. We had no idea what to expect—but we were immediately welcomed. Indeed, band leader Al Cobbs of the C. and J. Band would refer to "the Small's family" for the year and a half that the dances were held.

At Small's, we learned about things like breakfast dances

and Lindy contests; we saw shake dances and flash dancing. At Small's, musicians like James Moody and authors like Amiri Baraka would occasionally drop by. We met tap dancers like Buster Brown, Chuck Green, Honi Coles, and Cookie Cook. And one night in came Norma Miller with Frankie Manning in tow—which was how we met them for the first time. We began to realize just how important the Lindy and its originators were to New York's life and culture—and that it deserved to be more widely known and appreciated.

That is how the New York Swing Dance Society was formed. For when it became clear that Small's was once again going to close, our handful of regulars decided to try to keep the tradition of dancing to live big band music going. We knew that Al Minns had been taken to Sweden by a group called the Swedish Swing Society; I had even spent a week with them in Stockholm one summer while Al was there. So, early in 1985 a group of a dozen of us decided to form the New York Swing Dance Society. Our aim was to hold regular dances to big band music, to celebrate the contributions of the dance's originators.

It was in many ways a remarkable group. Few of us knew more about each other than our first names and what steps we did. It turned out that we had a wide range of occupations: a secretary, a lawyer, a chef, a university professor, a magazine editor. We never would have come in contact with each other but for this dance. Our ambition was hard to pull off—big bands are expensive, as are large, open dance floors. Fortunately, we found a place, the Cat Club, which agreed to give us a break on the rent on Sunday evenings.

Tragedy struck, however, when Al Minns was hospitalized in the spring of 1985. He was suffering from cancer of the esophagus, and he became incoherent. He died on April 25, ten days before the New York Swing Dance Society held its first dance. In the meantime, we had met several other original Lindy Hoppers, including Norma, Frankie, and ten or so others.

At the Cat Club, we had about a dozen bands which we rotated, including the C. and J. Band, the Harlem Blues and Jazz Band, the Loren Schoenberg Big Band, and many others. We occasionally had special events, such as Norma Miller's 70th birthday party, and from time to time hired special bands, like the Basie Band and Sun Ra Arkestra. The *New York Post* wrote that we were "the most thoroughly integrated club in Manhattan"; MTV said "It's a melting pot . . . the East Village meets Harlem." For many of us, the experience involved an entirely new exposure to music, dance, and African-American culture. I began to write about the dance and interview the old-timers.

We also learned about what had happened to Swing through the rest of the country. The dance had been transformed, and in different ways, depending on local conditions. The Carolinas had a languid, slowed-down version that had become known as the Shag. St. Louis had a fast version—the Imperial Style, they called it—that retained certain features of the old Charleston. Texas had two styles called the Push and the Whip. California was home to a version called the West Coast Swing. Not only were these different stylistically from each other and from the Lindy (or Savoy Style Swing, as some began to call it), but outside of New York, Swing clubs tended to emphasize competitions, while we tended to view our dances as social events.

Thanks to videos, personal contacts, and dance weekends

that became popular in the late 1980s, some of what we did here spread to the rest of the country, and some of what they did elsewhere became popular here. In 1989 I wound up in Cleveland for a night and noticed in a local paper an advertisement for a Swing dance. I hopped in the car and drove for half an hour, expecting to find the tired six-count Jitterbug step that at the time often passed for Swing dancing. Imagine my shock to see them doing an eight-count Lindy and fairly good swing-outs. I stopped and asked a woman where she had learned it. "George taught us," she said and pointed to someone in the corner. I went over to George and posed the question to him. "Oh, I learned that in a workshop in the hills of Pennsylvania," George said. "Big guy, by the name of Frankie Manning. Great dance. Everyone here likes it so we've mixed it in with what we're doing."

With all the contact between different Swing groups all over the country and with the assistance of the video camera Swing dancing is going through a major transition. There is a danger that the different styles will blend together into one homogenous style—a dance version of Esperanto. To keep the dance vital will be hard work. Even holding regular dances has proven extremely difficult for the New York Swing Dance Society, with costs of bands and dance spaces rising. And, as with other things that experience a renaissance, two opposing ideologies have emerged. For one, the dance should be preserved in its original, pristine form, like some folk dances are; for the other, the dance should be melded in with what the rest of the country is doing, making it more commercial. If either course were followed exclusively, the dance would die— the one because the dance would effectively be turned into a nostalgia trip, the other because the dance would lose its distinctiveness and capacity for personal expression. The New York Swing Dance Society is attempting to avoid both pitfalls by promoting the Savoy-style Lindy, while remaining open to other forms.

For a long time, the influence of the Lindy has been apparent in many African-American dance styles and even in the body movements of Latin dances and in Country-Western dance patterns. Recently, the Lindy has become more conspicuous thanks to films like *Stompin' at the Savoy*, *Malcolm X*, and pieces performed by Alvin Ailey and the American Ballroom Theater, choreographed by Norma Miller, with the assistance of Frankie Manning.

The New York Swing Dance Society hosted a special weekend Can't Top the Lindy Hop, on May 17–30, 1994, in celebration of Frankie Manning's 80th birthday. It drew hundreds of dancers from around the world. But even all of these events do not really measure the true influence of the Lindy. For how we dance, as Nietzsche knew and Plato suspected, has a lot to do with who we are. And every time we experience that smooth feeling that accompanies moving in synch with jazz music—that *Swing*—every time we do that, the Lindy has exerted its power over us.

Robert P. Crease
New York